Educatio
Southend
Westcliff-o
Essentials of Ocu
and The

23

?

Essentials of Ocular Pharmacology and Therapeutics

Kamal Kumar Sengupta, MS, DOMS
Research Associate, Eye Care & Research Centre, Kolkata
Formerly of the Pharmacology Department, North Bengal
University Medical College, District Darjeeling

and

Ranabir Mikherji, MS, DOMS, PhD, FRCOphth
Director, Eye Care & Research Centre, Kolkata
Formerly Professor and Head, Eye Department,
Calcutta National Medical College, Kolkata

Anshan

Anshan Limited, UK

Anshan Limited
6 Newlands Road
Tunbridge Wells
Kent TN4 9AT, UK
Tel/Fax: + 44(0) 1892 557767
E-mail: info@anshan.co.uk
Website: www.anshan.co.uk

Notice: Every effort has been made that the drug dosage schedules in this book are accurate and in accord with the standards accepted at the time of publication. However, the reader is urged to consult drug manufacturer's printed instructions, particularly regarding the recommended dose, indications and contraindications for administration and adverse reactions before administrating any of the drugs.

British Library Cataloguing in Publication Data
A catalogue record for this book is available from the British Library.

Not for sale in India, Pakistan and Bangladesh

ISBN-10: 1-905740-01-8
ISBN-13: 978-1-905740-01-7

This edition is co-published by B.I. Publications Pvt Ltd, New Delhi, India and Anshan Limited, Kent, UK, and printed at Saurabh Printers Pvt Ltd, Noida, India.

Preface

It is well known that a proper drug at proper time often saves the eye from almost inevitable blindness. On the other hand, at times many drugs used injudiciously may not only hasten blindness but also cause grave health hazards, including death. It is imperative that an ophthalmic practitioner like any other medical man must have fundamental knowledge of pharmacology and the drugs which he uses in his day to day practice. With this objective in view, we have compiled this book for ophthalmologists, optometrists, ophthalmic assistants, ophthalmic nurses and postgraduate students. Though we have endeavoured to make the book more practical-oriented for the clinicians, basic principles of the subject have also been incorporated which are expected to be beneficial for the students.

We are grateful to Dr. Suddhasatwya Chatterjee and Miss Panchali Mukherjee for their invaluable services in the preparation of the manuscript and to Mrs. Mandira Chakraborty for her excellent secretarial assistance.

We are thankful to the Publishers and their technical staff for their help in publishing the book.

Lastly, we shall feel rewarded if our objective is fulfilled and eye care professionals and also postgraduate students find this book a good compendium of a difficult but important subject.

Eye Care and Research Centre   Kamal Kumar Sengupta
Kolkata 700 017   Ranabir Mukherji

Acknowledgement

To make the book more authentic and up-to-date, we have freely collected materials from the standard text books on pharmacology and therapeutics and from many articles published in different books and journals. A list of such publications is given below. We express our indebtedness and sincere thanks to all authors and publishers.

1. Goodman & Gilmans. In: Hardman J.G., Limbird L.E, eds. *The Pharmacological Basis of Therapeutics.* 10th International edition. New York, USA: McGraw Hill Medical Publishing Division; 2001.
2. Tripathi K.D. *Essentials of Medical Pharmacology.* 5th ed. New Delhi, India: Jaypee Brothers Medical Publishers (P) Ltd.; 2003.
3. Levy R.H., Thummel K.E., Tranger W.F., Hansten P.D., Eichelbaum, M., eds. *Metabolic Drug Interactions.* Philadelphia, USA: Lippincott, Williams & Wilkins; 2000.
4. Scriver C.R., Beaudet A.L., Sly W.S., Valle D, eds. *The Metabolic and Molecular Basis of Inherited Diseases.* New York, USA: McGraw – Hill; 2000.
5. Mandell G.L., Bennett J.E., Dolin R., eds. *Mandell, Douglas and Bennett's Principle and Practice of Infectious Diseases.* 5th ed. Philadelphia, USA: Churchill Livingstone, Inc.; 2000.
6. Fechner P.U., Teichmann K.D. *Ocular Therapeutics – Pharmacology and Clinical Application.* 1st Indian ed. New Delhi, India: Jaypee Brothers; 1998.
7. Giacopini, ed. *Cholinesterase and Cholinesterase Inhibitors.* London: Martin Dunitz; 2000.

8.   Spencer P.S., Schauburd H.M., eds. *Experimental and Clinical Neurotoxicology.* 2nd ed. New York: Oxford University Press; 2000.

9.   Miller R.D., ed. *Anaesthesia.* 5th ed. Philadelphia, USA: Churchill Livingstone; 2000.

10. Seth S.D., ed. *Textbook of Pharmacology.* 2nd ed. New Delhi, India: B.I. Churchill Livingstone Pvt. Ltd.; 1999.

11. Satoskar R.S., Bhandarkar S.D., Ainapure S.S., *Pharmacology and Pharmacotherapeutics.* 6th ed. Mumbai, India: Popular Prakashan; 1999.

12. Vogelstein B, Kinzler K.W., eds. *The Genetic Basis of Human Cancer.* New York, USA: McGraw Hill; 1998

13. Albert D.M., Jalkobiec F.A., eds. *Principle and Practice of Ophthalmology: Clinical Practice,* Vols 4 and 5. Philadelphia, USA: Saunders; 1994.

14. Mitra A.K., ed. *Ophthalmic Drug Delivery System.* New York: Marcel Dekker; 1993.

In spite of our best intention, it is possible that inadvertently some names have been omitted in this list for which we would request them to accept this blanket acknowledgement.

Contents

CHAPTER 1

Introduction

Pharmacology is the study of the action of chemical substances, especially drugs on animals and humans. Systematic investigations of the effects of drugs started in the 19th century. The dawn of modern pharmacology began in 1849 when Rudolf Buchheim of Germany set up a pharmacology laboratory in the basement of his residence. From then onwards, pharmacology is recognized as a specialized discipline in medicine. The subject was further developed by Oswald Schmiedberg (1838-1921), a student of Buchheim, who is regarded as Founder of Modern Pharmacology. In India, Sir R.N. Chopra (1882-1973) is regarded as the 'Father of Modern Indian Pharmacology'. He will be ever remembered for his immortal work on indigenous drugs.

Pharmacology aims to unravel the mechanisms of the action of drugs in the living system and its scope is very wide. It includes the study of the action of drugs in a living body (pharmacodynamics), administration of drugs in treatment for disease (therapeutics), study of the source, composition, characteristics and preparation of drugs, study of poisons (toxicology), pharmaceutical chemistry, and the preparation and dispensing of drugs for medical use (pharmacy).

Some Definitions

Pharmacology: It is the science which deals with drugs (from the Greek 'Pharmacon' = drug; and 'Logos' = discourse in).
Drug: According to World Health Organization (WHO – 1966) "Drug is any substance or product that is used or intended to be used to modify or explore physiological systems or pathological states for the benefit of the recipient."

Pharmacokinetics: It means the chain of events that may occur in the body after the administration of a drug, i.e., (1) absorption, (2) distribution, (3) binding, (4) localization, (5) storage, (6) biotransformation and (7) excretion.

Example: Chloroquine is absorbed orally in sufficiently high amounts; about 50% of the absorbed amount gets bound to plasma, a portion gets tightly bound to nuclear chromatin and melanin. It is concentrated in lungs, liver, kidney, spleen, retina, etc., partly metabolized by liver and partly excreted in urine and has a $t_{1/2}$ of approximately 3-10 days.

Pharmacodynamics: Pharmacodynamics means the biochemical and physiological action of a drug on the body. It also includes the mechanism of action of the drug.

Example: Benzodiazepines facilitate GABA action but they do not possess GABA-mimetic action and this is actually the low ceiling CNS depressive mechanism of action of benzodiazepines.

Ocular pharmacology: It is a part of clinical pharmacology which deals with detailed scientific analysis of the action of a drug in human volunteers to explore its practical implications in a clinical condition.

Essential drugs: According to WHO essential drugs are: "Those that satisfy the healthcare needs of the majority of population." Therefore, it is evident that such drugs should be available at all times in adequate amounts and in appropriate dosage forms. WHO published in 1977 a model list of essential drugs. Government of India has published its own model list of 279 essential drugs in 1996.

Orphan drugs: These drugs are required for the management, prevention and diagnosis of a rare clinical condition. The production costs of such drugs are high and are usually not recovered from the sales. A few examples of this group of drugs are liothyronin, calcitonin, protamine sulfate, etc.

Chronopharmacology and chronobiotics: Chronopharmacology refers to a particular biological rhythm occurring in the body after taking a drug.

Example: Bronchospasm induced by histamine occurs at midnight, while bronchospasm caused by acetylcholine occurs in the evening.

Chronobiotics are substances which reset the biological clock (circadian rhythm) of the body, if it is disturbed. Melatonin of pineal gland has a role in regulation of circadian rhythm. Circadian rhythm is found to be disturbed in intercontinental travelers who travel by Jet planes. This is called Jet lag, which occurs due to confusion created by disturbances in the normal day and night cycle to which the subject is usually accustomed. The disturbance can be prevented by consuming a 3 mg tablet of melatonin prior to taking an intercontinental flight.

Pharmacy: It deals with the art and science of preparation of various forms of drugs or various combinations of drugs in suitable proportions and suitable dosage forms meant for administration into the living system. Some of the important aspects of pharmacy are cultivation of medicinal plants, isolation of active ingredients, chemical analysis and bio-standardization of products thus obtained, synthesis of new chemical molecules, studies on their structure-activity relationship (SAR), etc.

Toxicology: This science deals with poisons. Poisons are substances which endanger life and many drugs in high doses act as poisons. Toxicology deals with clinical manifestations, diagnosis, management and preventive aspect of poisons and poisoning.

Pharmacometrics: Each and every drug can be qualitatively and quantitatively studied for its pharmacological activity utilizing techniques like chemical assay, bio-assay, immuno-assay, etc. The branch of pharmacology dealing with these studies is called pharmacometrics.

Pharmacogenetics: It is a science which deals with influence of genetic pattern on the metabolic process of a drug. Example: The concentration of atropine required to dilate the pupil in cases of black race is more and in cases of blue irides it is less.

Pharmacoeconomics: It is a topic of current interest. India is a poor country and a medical practitioner should prescribe a treatment schedule keeping the following facts in mind.

   (a) Unnecessary medication should be avoided.

   (b) A drug should be prescribed in generic name, as it is less costly.

   (c) Unnecessary investigations for academic interest should be avoided. Drug-drug interaction with undesirable iatrogenic manifestations should be kept in mind.

   (d) Before prescribing a costly treatment schedule, a medical practitioner should have a clear idea of the outcome of the procedure.

Pharmaco-epidemiology: After a drug comes to the market it has to pass through phase IV or the post- marketing surveillance phase. This process is also called pharmaco-vigilance. Opinion is collected, particularly regarding adverse reactions of a drug, from a large number of medical practitioners who have used it. The basic idea behind pharmaco-vigilance is to prevent human sufferings due to the use of a drug.

A long-term project is undertaken to know the actual effect of a drug in the management of a particular condition. These studies are called pharmaco-epidemiological studies. Such studies are conducted both as prospective cohort studies (based on 10-15 years forward-looking observations) and retrospective cohort studies (based on 10-30 years observations of past records).

Sources of Drugs

Important sources of drugs are as follows:
1. *Vegetable kingdom*: Pilocarpine (obtained from leaves of pilocarpus microphyllus), atropine (obtained from leaves of atropa belladonna), etc.
2. *Animal kingdom:* Insulin (usually obtained from pig's pancreas).
3. *Mineral kingdom*: Iron (used as antianaemics)
4. *Microbes:* Antibiotics (penicillins from penicillium chrysogenum), enzyme (streplokinase from streptococci), etc.
5. *Synthetic origin:* Presently most of the drugs used in medical practice are of synthetic origin, e.g., Corticosteroids, NSAIDs, etc.
6. *Human origin*: Immunoglobulins, growth hormone, etc.
7. *Products of recombinant DNA technology:* Human insulin, interferon alpha 2a and alpha 2b, etc.

Drug Development

There are many routes to development of new drug molecules. Of these, the following need consideration by a clinician.

Screening Technique

Various chemicals of plant or animal origin are studied systematically for their pharmacological properties. Drugs like meprobamate, methaqualone, etc., were discovered by this technique.

Utilizing SAR (Structure-Activity Relationship)

Structure of a chemical is related to its pharmacological properties and hence a change in structure may lead to change in these properties. Replacement of a chemical moiety present at a particular position in a chemical structure of a known drug by some other chemical radical and then studying its pharmacological properties is an important method of newer drug development. For example, the earlier H-1 antagonists were prepared by substituting ethylamine side chain attached to the imidazole ring of histamine.

Laboratory Synthesis Based On Clinical Observations

When sulfanilamide was discovered it was found to possess mild diuretic property. Based on this observation, various compounds were synthesized and ultimately breakthrough came with the introduction of chlorothiazide diuretic, which was launched as the first orally effective and reliable diuretic.

Accidental Discovery

Probably all major discoveries are accidental to some extent. The classical example is that of the accidental discovery of penicillin in 1928 by Sir Alexander Fleming, who was actually studying microbiological aspects of staphylococci.

Utilizing Recombinant DNA Technology/Genetic Engineering

This is a modern method of producing drugs. Classical example is production of human insulin by recombinant DNA technology in *Escherichia coli*. Pharmacologically genetic engineering technology is utilized for gene modification and genre transfer. However, this science is still in its infancy but work is going on at a very high speed.

Testing

Before a drug molecule is ready for use it has to undergo a series of animal experiments and human clinical trials. Following steps are involved in testing a drug:

Animal testing

1. First step in animal studies consists of acute toxicity studies.
2. Second step is to carry out long-term toxicity studies.
3. Third step involves observations on the reproductive system.
4. Fourth step is determination of mutagenic and carcinogenic potentialities of the test drug.

After all the four steps are complete and if the drug is thought to be suitable for human trials, it has to pass through four phases of human trial.

Human trials

1. Phase I human clinical trial is conducted on a selected number of volunteers.
2. If the preliminary report of the test drug is satisfactory, Phase II clinical trial is started on a large number of patients.
3. Phase III studies are most important. Phase III is also called controlled clinical trial, which means comparative study of test drug therapy versus previously established drug therapy or placebo therapy, under standardized conditions. The test performed is 100% double blind control trial study. From Phase I to Phase III, clinical trial takes about six years. In India, data of all these phases are submitted to Drug Controller General of Govt. of India, who, if satisfied by the data, issues permission for open market survey, i.e., Phase IV.
4. Phase IV is also called post-marketing surveillance phase, where many clinicians use the drug on patients and data regarding any additional toxicity or additional therapeutic use are collected. For example, acetazolamide was introduced as a diuretic, but soon its antiglaucoma effect was recognized.

In this way an unknown drug molecule after passing through all these stages earns reputation and ultimately becomes a trusted therapeutic agent.

Drug Assay

It means determination of the potency of a drug molecule in a unit quantity of preparation. Such assays can be done chemically, biologically and immunologically.

Chemical Assay

The common techniques used are high-pressure liquid chromatography, spectrophotometry, mass spectrometry, gas chromatography, fluorometry, etc. When aminoglycoside antibiotics are used under compulsive ophthalmic condition in a patient with renal dysfunction, estimation of blood level of the drug helps to keep the patient out of danger.

Bioassay

It is used in cases where chemical assay methodology is not possible, e.g., estimation of LATS, prostaglandin, hypothalamic factors controlling anterior pituitary, etc.

Immunoassay

This method is mainly utilized for hormone assay. RIA (radioimmunoassay) is widely practiced. More recent advancements in the field of drug assay include radio receptor assay, ELISA (enzyme linked immunosorbent assay) and IRMA (immunoradiometric assay).

Nomenclature of Drugs

A drug is usually identified by three names:
- By class, e.g., Nonsteroidal anti-inflammatory agent.
- By non-proprietary name, e.g., Ibuprofen.
- By proprietary name, e.g., Brufen.

In addition, every drug has a chemical name according to its chemical structure.

Important Sources of Information on Drugs

Pharmacopoeia: It is a book which contains the accepted standards for drugs and medicinal preparations with their recommended doses.

Examples: British Pharmacopoeia (BP), Indian Pharmacopoeia (IP), etc.

National Formulary, British National Formulary (BNF) and National Formulary (NF) of India: These are published by American Pharmaceutical Association, British Medical Association and the Pharmaceutical Society of Great Britain, and Government of India, respectively. They contain detailed information about all products available in the country concerned.

British Pharmaceutical Codex: It is yet another publication by pharmaceutical society of Great Britain which in addition to product information gives some additional important information like standard of purity of a substance that is not provided in British Pharmacopoeia.

AMA Drug evaluations: It is published by American Medical Association council of drugs, which gives a neutral opinion about individual drugs and their comparative study with other drugs of the same group. The information provided is always current in nature.

CHAPTER 2

Routes of Administration of Drugs

In general, the major routes of administration of drugs in human body are topical, enteral, paraenteral, sublingual, pulmonary and rectal.

Routes of Administration of Drugs for Eye Diseases

The two important routes of drug administration in the case of eye diseases are:
- Systemic route
- Local route

Systemic Route

The systemic route includes drug administration through oral route and by injections. There are certain barriers affecting the entrance of drug inside the eye when the drug is used through systemic route. Two such important barriers are: (i) blood aqueous barrier and (ii) blood retinal barrier.

(i) Blood aqueous barrier: The non-pigmented layer of ciliary epithelium and endothelium of iris vessels constitute this barrier. This barrier is said to have tight junctions of leaky type.

(ii) Blood retinal barrier: This is believed to be situated in retinal pigment epithelium and endothelium of retinal blood vessels. This barrier is said to have tight junctions of non-leaky type.

There are some other factors that modify the entrance of drug inside the eye. Out of the various factors, two factors worth mentioning are: (i) lipid solubility of the drug molecule and (ii) molecular size of the drug concerned. Such factors are responsible for the fact that sulfonamides can attain much higher concentrations in aqueous humour compared to penicillin.

But whenever there is an inflammation, the effectivity of all such factors and barriers is lost. So, during acute inflammation, penicillin can also attain a very high concentration inside the ocular tissues.

Penetration of drugs through cornea

When a drug is given in drop or ointment form, it has to penetrate cornea to reach the anterior chamber. Corneal epithelium allows lipid soluble drugs and stroma allows water-soluble drugs to enter inside anterior chamber. So, drugs which are both lipid and water-soluble attain maximum concentration in aqueous. It has been observed that destruction of epithelium enhances the permeability of drug and hence epithelium can be considered as main barrier influencing entrance of drug inside the eye by topical route.

Local Route

Local route includes eye drops, eye ointment, ocusert, drug impregnated contact lens, subconjunctival injection, subtenon injection, retrobulbar injection, and injection into the eye (i) intracameral – in aqueous and (ii) intravitreal – in the vitreous body.

Eye drops

The conjunctival sac can retain only one drop at a time and so only one drop of drug is enough and it is economical too. Problems with eye drops are that they are quickly drained out of eye through naso-lacrimal passage and the concentration of drug also gets diluted by tear film.

According to the current concepts, the retaining capacity of conjunctival sac is 20 to 30 microlitre when the eyes are kept open while the normal volume of tear is approximately 7 to 10 microlitre. The eye drops used are of two types: (a) small eye drop (5 to 20 microlitre) and (b) conventional large eye drop (30 to 70 microlitre). Small eye drop is usually preferred as it is economical.

- Preservatives like benzalkonium cause temporary loss of integrity of corneal epithelium and help penetration of drugs like topical beta-blockers. But it may cause corneal irritation.

- When an eye drop contains drug in suspension form, the optimum size should be 2 micrometer.
- Vehicles of the eye drop which increase the contact time of drug molecule are hydroxymethylcellulose, polyvinyl alcohol, polyvinyl pyrolidone, etc.

Eye ointment

It is superior to eye drop as it stays in conjunctival sac for a longer period and its drainage through nasolacrimal duct is minimum. It is particularly useful for children where systemic absorption of the concerned drug from nasal and stomach mucous membrane may have adverse effects. However, there are two main disadvantages of eye ointment: (i) it cannot be used during daytime as it causes hazy vision and (ii) sometimes the ointment base may cause allergic reactions.

Ocusert

It is a device through which a particular concentration of drug is released and absorbed through conjunctiva at a particular rate throughout the day and night and the effect persists for a few days. The classical example is pilocarpine ocusert used in the treatment of glaucoma.

Contact lens soaked in drug

Sometimes a drug is soaked in a soft contact lens and placed over cornea and there is continuous release of drug, which is absorbed through cornea.

Retrobulbar injection

The best example of this method of drug administration is retrobulbar lignocaine injection for producing ciliary block during cataract operation.

Subconjunctival or subtenon injection

The usual drugs administered through this route are steroids, antibiotics, atropine, etc., for various ophthalmic conditions like iritis, corneal ulcer, etc. Through this route, the drug attains a very high concentration inside the eye and the level is also maintained for a longer period. It is interesting to note that although the injection is given in subconjunctival tissue, the absorption occurs through cornea.

Direct injection into the eye

The classical example of this method is antibiotic injection into vitreous cavity in endophthalmitis.

CHAPTER 3

Pharmacokinetics

Pharmacokinetics is the study of the process by which a drug is absorbed, distributed, metabolized and eliminated by the body. It includes stages of absorption of the drug, its distribution, binding to plasma and tissue proteins, storage, biotransformation and ultimately excretion from the body. For all these things to happen, the drug molecule has to cross a barrier, called plasma membrane. Of course, in case of intravenous injection, the drug does not have to cross such a biological membrane. The pharmacokinetic process is illustrated in Fig. 3.1.

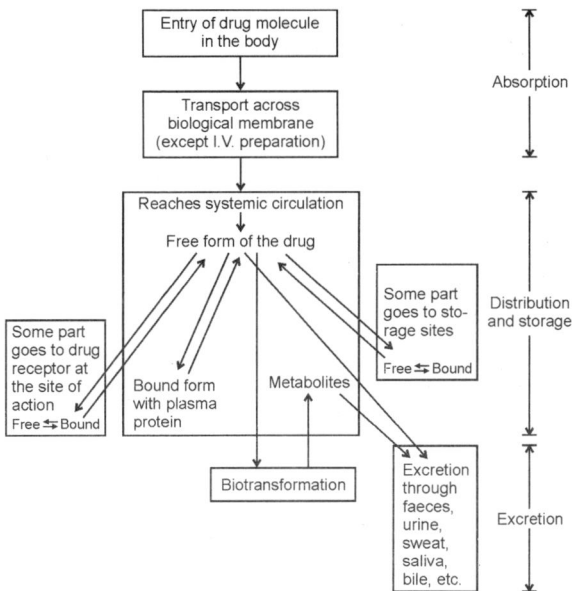

Fig. 3.1. The pharmacokinetic process

Transport across the Cell Membrane

The cell membrane (approximately 100 A° thick) is a semipermeable bilipid layer (phospholipid and cholesterol) in which the proteins are embedded or floating at variable depths. One portion of the lipid is hydrophilic, while the other portion is hydrophobic. It has been observed that some proteins traverse through the whole thickness of membrane (trans-membrane proteins), which possess channels for diffusion. Glutamic acid content is found to be high in the protein layers of plasma membrane. Some of the protein molecules of outer layer have connections with branched polysaccharides. The terminal residues of these polysaccharides are negatively charged sialic acid. The proteins situated in hydrophobic zones of lipid bilayer are found to be rich in leucine.

The drug passes through this membrane by:

(i) a passive transport mechanism (which involves simple diffusion and filtration), or,

(ii) a specialized transport mechanism (which involves carrier transport mechanism and process of pinocytosis).

Passive Transport Mechanism

(a) Simple diffusion

This is the most common process of transport, which does not require any energy mechanism or carrier system. The flow occurs from higher to lower concentration. The rate of flow is governed by lipid-water partition coefficient of the drug. The drugs which possess high lipid-water partition coefficient are absorbed at a higher rate.

In this process, two important factors—pH and degree of ionization—also play a vital role. Acidic drugs like aspirin are absorbed better from stomach and the basic drugs like atropine are absorbed better from intestine.

(b) Filtration

In this process, water-soluble drugs can pass through aqueous pores in plasma membrane or via paracellular spaces. The best example of filtration process is the glomerular filtration process, which is an important mechanism for excretion of the majority of drugs. Here, size of the pores in the plasma membrane is the most important factor. Most of the cells of human body have small pores of approximately 4 A° which allow drugs having molecular weight not more than 100 to 200 to pass through. But capillaries have larger pores, about 40 A° (except capillaries of brain) and so larger-size drug molecules can easily pass through them. But passage of drugs through capillaries mostly depends on the rate of blood flow, as in glomerular filtration.

Specialized Transport Mechanism

Carrier transport mechanism

Carriers are specialized type of membrane proteins, called transporters. When such type of transport requires energy (when the movement of drug molecule occurs against the concentration gradient) the term used is *active transport* and when energy is not required (when the movement occurs along the concentration gradient) the term used is *facilitated diffusion*. When energy is required it is derived from ATP. The example of facilitated diffusion is uptake of glucose by the cells and the example of active transport is absorption of levodopa.

Pinocytosis

In this process a drug molecule is engulfed by the cell and is transported across by formation of vesicles. Usually, protein molecules and larger drug molecules are transported in this way.

First Pass Metabolism and Bioavailability

First Pass Metabolism

It is a phenomenon of drug metabolism. When a drug is swallowed, it reaches liver after absorption by the digestive system. The liver metabolizes many drugs and in some cases only a small amount of unchanged drug enters the systemic circulation and, therefore, the bioavailability of the drug is reduced. The intravenous and intramuscular routes avoid the first pass effect. For example, some drugs like isosorbide dinitrate or glyceryl trinitrate (used for urgent coronary

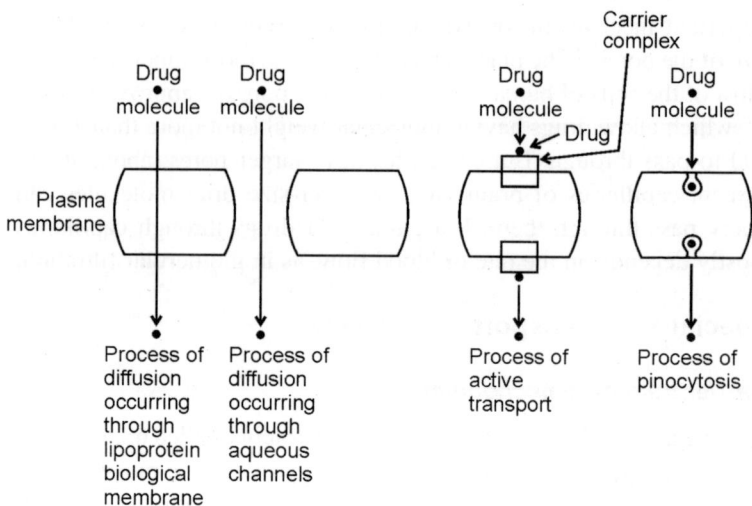

Fig. 3.2. Schematic representation of carriage of drug molecule across the biological membrane

dilatation in acute angina), when given orally are subjected to first pass metabolism by liver and the oral bioavailability achieved is not up to the desired level. But if the same drug is given sublingually, it can by-pass the liver induced first pass metabolism and can act on target tissue within a few minutes. However, only lipid soluble and non-irritant drugs can be administered through sublingual route.

Bioavailability

According to FDA (United States Food and Drug Administration), bioavailability is defined as "The rate and extent to which the therapeutic moiety is absorbed and becomes available to the site of drug action". When a drug is given by intravenous route, the bioavailability is 100%. But the bioavailability is decreased when the drug is given by oral route. Multiple factors like local binding of the drugs to tissues, first pass metabolism, pharmaceutical factors, etc., have been held responsible for this phenomenon. However, pharmaceutical factors seem to be the most important and affect bioavailability.

Distribution

After a drug reaches systemic circulation, it is distributed to various tissues and ultimately reaches its target tissue, i.e., the site of action. But this process is not so simple, as the drug has to cross many barriers, some portion gets bound to plasma protein, and some portion goes to specific tissue binding sites, etc. Other important factors which play an important role in the distribution of a drug are regional vascularity, redistribution, lipid solubility, ionization at the local pH, dissociation constant of the drug, size of drug molecule, chemical structure of the drug and, lastly, the pathological status of the patient concerned.

Barriers Concerned with Distribution Process

The most important barriers are:
- Blood-brain barrier
- Blood-CSF barrier
- Enzymatic blood-brain barrier
- Placental barrier

In the substance of brain, the endothelial cells of capillaries have tight junctions with absence of intercellular pores of larger size. In addition, a glial cell envelope covers the capillaries. This is called *blood-brain barrier.* Similarly, in choroid plexus the capillaries are lined by special type of epithelium which has tight junctions and it is called *blood-CSF barrier.* A special barrier called *enzymatic blood-brain barrier* also exists which restricts the entry of some neurotransmitters like acetylcholine, catecholamines, etc., inside the brain substance in active form. Blood-brain barrier is absent in some parts of brain like chemoreceptor trigger zone, and some paraventricular areas. Usually, the lipid-soluble drugs are allowed to enter through blood-brain and blood-CSF barriers. During an acute inflammatory process, the permeability of barriers increases and even non-lipid soluble drugs gain entry through these barriers. As far as the exit of the drug from brain or CSF is concerned, the drug is driven out by bulk flow of CSF through arachnoid villi.

The placental barrier is an incomplete barrier. Any drug given to mother in high concentrations for a prolonged period reaches the fetus in appreciable amounts.

Plasma Protein Binding

Acidic drugs (e.g. NSAIDs, benzodiazepines, etc.) bind to plasma albumin and basic drugs (e.g. Lignocaine, beta blockers, etc.) bind to alpha one acid glycoprotein.

Tissue Binding

Some drugs exhibit increased affinity for special cellular constituent, so much so that such binding may cause local tissue toxicity, e.g., chloroquine may produce chloroquine retinopathy.

Tissue Perfusion

If a highly lipid soluble drug like thiopentone sodium is given intravenously, there is immediate high rise of concentration of the drug in brain (as brain has good tissue perfusion) and the individual becomes unconscious but the effect lasts for very small period of time because the less well perfused tissue like muscle (fat content of muscle is quite high) continue to absorb the drug. This phenomenon is called *redistribution.*

Influence of Fatty Tissue

Some important drugs are concentrated in fatty tissue, e.g., minocycline. When the level of free drug in plasma falls, there is mobilization of drug from fatty tissue depots and the plasma level of the free drug is again quickly restored.

Biotransformation

Biotransformation is a process in which lipid-soluble substances are converted into lipid-insoluble substances, which are then excreted from the body. Substances which have molecular weight less than 300 are excreted in urine and those having molecular weight more than 300 are excreted in faeces via bile. Biotransformation process involves two types of reactions: phase I (non-synthetic reactions) and phase II (synthetic reactions). Metabolites of phase I reactions may be excreted or may undergo phase II reaction (depending on nature of metabolite). Some drugs may directly undergo phase II reactions and the metabolites are excreted. Some non-lipid soluble drugs (e.g. Streptomycin) are excreted as such without undergoing biotransformation reactions. Some drugs undergo molecular rearrangement in plasma and are excreted without any help of the drug metabolizing enzyme system. Such type of metabolism of the drug is called Hofmann elimination (e.g. Atracurium – a skeletal muscle relaxant). The process of biotransformation will be clear from the following chart (Fig.3.3)

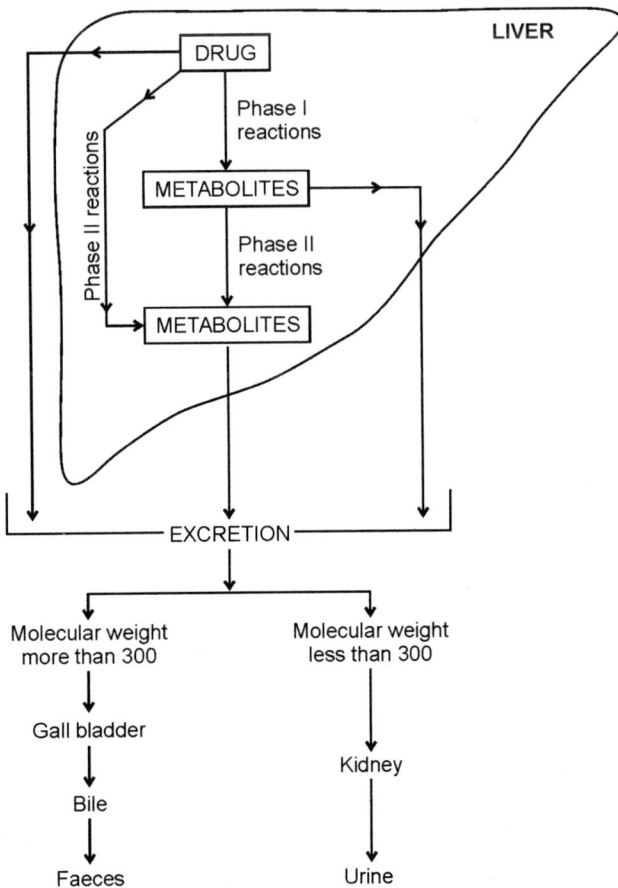

Fig. 3.3. Schematic representation of the biotransformation process

The main site of biotransformation process is liver. Other sites are plasma, kidney, intestine and lungs. In general, metabolites of phase I may be either active or inactive but the metabolites of phase II reactions are usually inactive. Some drugs may be pharmacologically inert as such but become active after biotransformation. Examples of such drugs used in ophthalmology are dipivefrine (converted to epinephrine) and valacyclovir (converted to acyclovir). Such drugs are called *Pro-drugs*

Important phase I reactions are oxidation, reduction, hydrolysis, cyclization and decyclization. Some of the important examples are:

Oxidation	–	Phenacetin to paracetamol.
Reduction	–	Nitro reduction of chloramphenicol.
Hydrolysis	–	Procaine to procainamide
Cyclization	–	Proguanil
Decyclization	–	Barbiturates

Important phase II reactions are:

Glucuronide conjugation	–	e.g. chloramphenicol
Sulfate conjugation	–	e.g. paracetamol
Glycine conjugation	–	e.g. acetyl salicylic acid.
Acetylation	–	e.g. isoniazide
Glutathione conjugation	–	e.g. naphthalene

Enzymes Related to Metabolism of Drugs

These enzymes are divided into two major groups: Microsomal and non-microsomal enzymes.

Microsomal enzymes

These are situated mainly on smooth endoplasmic reticulum of liver. They are also found in kidneys, lungs, and intestinal mucous membrane. Important examples of this group of enzyme system are glucuronyl transferase, monooxygenases, and cytochrome P-450. This enzyme system is inducible by various drugs (e.g. phenytoin, rifampicin, barbiturates, etc.), food (charcoal-broiled meat) and tobacco smoke. Microsomal enzyme system is involved in majority of the oxidation, reduction, hydrolysis, glucuronide conjugation, etc., type of biochemical reactions. Induction of enzyme means increase in synthesis of enzymes (but there is no activation of latent enzymes or enzyme precursors). Tobacco smoke increases the metabolism of theophylline (by enzyme induction) and hence the condition of bronchial asthma worsens. Similarly, phenytoin may cause failure of oral contraceptives by increasing its metabolic degradation.

Non-microsomal enzymes

Non-microsomal enzyme system is located mainly in the cytoplasm and mitochondria of liver cells. They are also present in many other organs including plasma. Important members of this group are amidase, conjugase, esterase, etc. This enzyme system is mainly involved in all conjugations (except glucuronide conjugation), hydrolytic reaction and some of the oxidation-reduction reactions. This enzyme system is non inducible.

Both microsomal and nonmicrosomal enzymes can be inhibited. Such enzyme inhibition processes have been utilized in therapeutics for management of various diseases. A few important examples are:

- Inhibition of carbonic anhydrase by acetazolamide, dorzolamide, etc., is utilized in the management of glaucoma.
- Inhibition of cyclo-oxygenase (COX) by majority of NSAIDs is utilized in the various inflammatory conditions of eye.
- Inhibition of angiotensin II converting enzyme (ACE) by enalapril is utilized in the management of hypertension.

Excretion

The drug or its metabolites are excreted through renal channel, biliary channel, pulmonary channel, sweat, saliva and milk.

- Water-soluble substances of molecular weight less than 300 are excreted through renal channel. Aminoglycoside antibiotics are excreted in unchanged form by glomerular filtration. Alkaline urine facilitates removal of NSAIDs and acidic urine facilitates removal of beta blockers by modifying tubular reabsorption mechanism. Penicillin is excreted by tubular secretion.
- Drugs or metabolites of molecular weight more than 300 are excreted through biliary channel, mainly as glucuronide conjugate.

- Anaesthetic gases and ethanol are usually excreted through pulmonary channel.

Drugs like rifampicin, clofazimine, etc., are excreted through sweat, saliva and tears. And so these secretions may be stained orange red due to rifampicin or reddish black due to clofazimine.

Most of the drugs are excreted in nominal amount in milk. But some of the drugs, excreted via milk, are regarded as potentially toxic, e.g., tetracycline, amiodarone, sulfasalazine, etc.

Elimination Kinetics

Most drugs are subjected to metabolic degradation in such a way that a constant fraction of drug present in the plasma is metabolized in unit time. If plasma concentration is increased, the metabolism is also increased proportionately per unit time. So, such type of elimination is dependant on plasma concentration and drugs following such type of kinetics are said to follow first order (exponential) kinetics.

But there are some drugs which do not follow the above principle. In case of these drugs, the rate of elimination remains constant with time and elevation of plasma concentration does not lead to increase in metabolism. Such drugs are said to follow zero order (saturation) kinetics. So, in this case whatever may be the plasma concentration only a fixed amount of the drug is eliminated in unit time. In zero order kinetics, if the dose (i.e., plasma concentration) is increased, the plasma half life also increases and this may lead to unpredictable or even toxic manifestation of the concerned drug. Classical examples of the drugs following saturation kinetics (zero order kinetics) are ethyl alcohol, dicoumarol, heparin, phenytoin, etc. Zero order kinetics is believed to be due to lack of availability of drug metabolizing enzyme system.

Clearance

Clearance is an important pharmacokinetical concept, which is useful in determining the quantity of drug required to keep up a steady state in the system. Clearance of a drug means the volume of blood or plasma completely cleared of that particular drug in unit time. Mathematically, it can be expressed as:

Clearance = Rate of elimination of a particular drug/ plasma concentration of that drug.

Half Life (t ₁/₂)

A drug, after administration in the system, reaches its peak value after full absorption. Then there is a sharp fall for sometime due to distribution of the drug. After this, there is slow declining phase due to elimination of the drug. If a drug follows first order elimination kinetics, the half life or plasma half life (t $_{1/2}$) is regarded as the time required for the plasma level to reduce to half. This is a very important parameter by which a clinician understands the behaviour pattern of a drug so that the dose schedule may be adjusted accordingly to get maximum therapeutic benefit. From bioavailability study curves, by plotting log plasma concentration against time, plasma half life can be easily determined. If drug is given I.V., which follows first order kinetics of elimination (and assuming it to behave as one-compartment model of distribution), the plot shows an initial sharp fall phase due to distribution (also called alpha phase)and then a slow sustained declining phase due to elimination (also called beta phase).

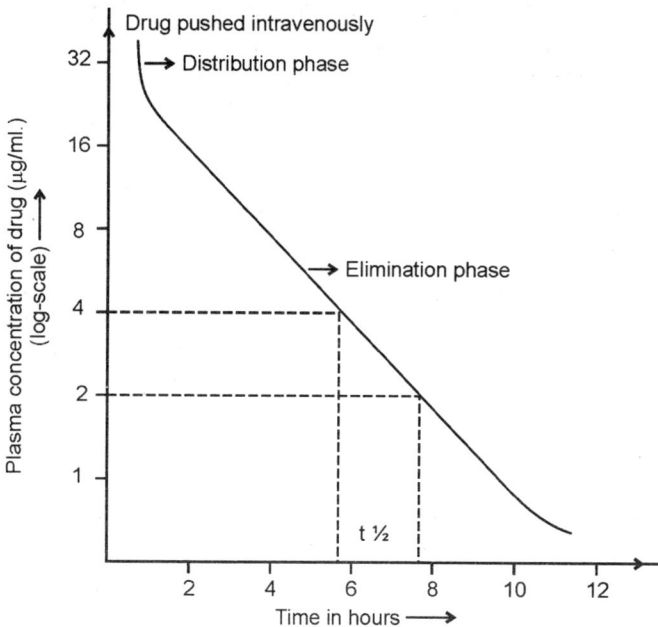

Fig. 3.4. A semilog plasma concentration-time plot of a drug administered intravenously and having a rapid one compartment distribution and first order elimination kinetics

Mathematically, $t_{1/2}$ is directly proportional to volume of distribution of the drug and is inversely proportional to its clearance. It is represented by the following equation:

$t_{1/2} = 0.693 \times V/Cl$, where V is volume and Cl is clearance.

In connection with half life, three important terms are commonly used: plasma half life, elimination half life and biological effect half life.

Plasma half life: It is the time during which the concentration of a drug in plasma gets reduced to half.

Elimination half life (also called Biological half life): It is the time required for half the quantity of a drug deposited in a living organism to be metabolized or eliminated by normal biological processes. In other words, it is the time during which the amount of drug present in the system, after attaining equilibrium with plasma and other compartments (viz. muscles, fats etc.), is reduced to half. Radioisotope technology is used to measure this half life.

Biological effect (half life): It is the time during which the pharmacological effect of a particular drug (or its metabolite) declines to half. Classical examples are 'hit and run' drugs where the pharmacological effect persists long after the drug has disappeared from the plasma, viz., reserpine, MAO inhibitors, antineoplastic drugs, etc.

Concept of steady state or 'plateau' principle

By knowing half life, one can assess the time required by a drug to reach steady state concentration in blood. Steady state means when the concentration of drug in plasma fluctuates between C_{max} (maximum concentration) and C_{min} (minimum concentration) represented by peak and trough respectively as shown in Fig. 3.5. To reach the steady state, at least 4 to 5 half lives are required.

Methods for Prolongation of the Action of a Drug

In the modern life style, full of stress and strain, prolongation of drug action is an important issue as a long acting drug (to be administered only once a day) is appreciated and accepted by the majority of patients. From the pharmacological point of view, drugs which have $t_{1/2}$ of 4

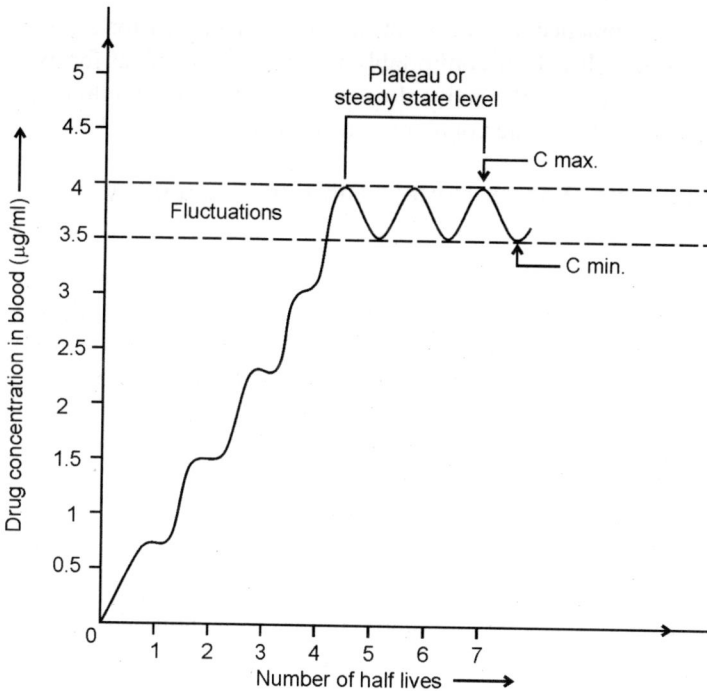

Fig. 3.5. Diagram illustrating steady state concentration (plateau) on repeated administration of a drug orally

hours or less are suitable for long acting drug formulation technology. But there is no point of prolonging the drug action of medicines which already have $t_{1/2}$ of 12 hours or more. Now, some important commonly used methods adopted to prolong drug action are as follows:

Delaying Absorption of a Drug Molecule

Some of the important technologies in this regard are sustained release tablet formulations, spansules, hydrodynamically balanced drug delivery system (HBS), amalgamation of a protein in drug molecule, esterification of a drug, biodegradable and non-biodegradable implantation technology, etc.

Some ultramodern technologies are transdermal drug delivery system, ocusert, osmotic pump device etc. Of these, ocusert is popular in ophthalmic practice as a constant rate delivery system for a drug like pilocarpine. It is kept comfortably in lower conjunctival fornix. In pilocarpine ocusert, the active drug is placed in between ethylene vinyl and ethylene acetate copolymer membranes.

Increasing the Plasma Protein Binding Capacity of a Drug by Chemical Manipulation

Examples of such drugs are ultra-long acting sulphonamides (sulfadoxine, sulfamethoxypyrazine, etc.) and suramin sodium (a trypanocidal drug having activity against Onchocerca volvulus). Ultra-long acting sulfonamides are effective up to 7 days after administration ($t_{1/2}$ = 5 to 9 days) and a single I.V. administration of suramin sodium can be detected in plasma even up to three months.

Suppressing the Biotransformation of the Drug Molecule

A classical example is inhibition of hydrolysis of imipenem (a recent broad spectrum beta lactam antibiotic) by dehydropeptidase I (found in brush borders of renal tubular cells), by cilastatin (which increases the therapeutic efficacy of the former).

Suppressing the Renal Excretion of a Drug by Utilizing the Principle of Drug-Drug Interaction

One of the classical examples of this method is inhibition of secretion of penicillin and ampicillin by renal tubular cells by probenecid and thus prolonging the action, which is particularly useful in the management of conditions like subacute bacterial endocarditis and gonorrhoea.

CHAPTER 4

Pharmacodynamics–Gene Based Therapy and Adverse Drug Reactions (ADR)

Pharmacodynamics is the study of the mechanism by which the drug produces a response. It also deals with various types of drug interactions. Drugs can never produce a new function in the body (except gene based therapy). Under normal circumstances drugs can produce stimulation (e.g. pilocarpine stimulates sphincter pupillae), depression (e.g. alcohol depresses CNS), substitution (e.g. replacement therapy in Addison's disease), cytotoxic action (e.g. antineoplastics), irritation (e.g. purgatives irritate gastro intestinal tract) and modification of immunological status of the system (e.g. immunosuppressives).

Mechanism of Action of a Drug

A drug may act through:
- Its physical properties, e.g., adsorption, osmotic property, radioactivity, radio-opaque property, etc.
- Chemical action, e.g., neutralization of gastric acidity by antacids, chelation of iron by desferrioxamine, etc.
- Action on primary drug targets, like receptors
- By enzyme inhibition, e.g., acetazolamide reduces IOP by inhibiting carbonic anhydrase.

Receptors

Receptors are dynamic, functional macromolecular components of a cell, protein in nature, situated either on the surface of cell or in the cytoplasm or inside the nucleus.

- Interaction of various hormones, autacoids neuro-transmitters and drug molecules with receptor produces physiological or pharmacological response.

Some special types of receptors

(a) **Spare receptors**. It is postulated that even when a receptor is blocked by irreversible blocker, an agonist is still capable of producing undiminished maximum response. For example, if beta adrenergic receptors are blocked irreversibly and then adrenaline is pushed, there is still production of an undiminished maximum inotropic response. So, spare receptors are explored only in presence of antagonist.

(b) **Silent receptors**. A drug when bound to such receptors, exhibits no pharmacological response. Examples of such receptors are plasma protein (where a portion of drug gets bound) and silent tissue receptors. The concept of silent receptor explains the phenomenon of tolerance and withdrawal phenomenon. A drug after prolonged use usually blocks the receptors present in a target organ. Now on increasing the dose, the pharmacological effect is perceived due to activation of silent receptors. When the drug is withdrawn, these silent receptors plus the normal receptors of target organ (which are now devoid of the drug) induce a state of withdrawal syndrome as the number of functioning receptors is increased leading to rebound hyperactive phenomenon.

(c) **Presynaptic receptors**. Such receptors are usually found in axonal terminals (may be presyanaptic or prejunctional). They may also be found on cell bodies of neurons. If these receptors are stimulated, usually there occurs an inhibitory response due to inhibition of release of excitatory neurotransmitter. Example: Noradrenaline, an endogenous transmitter, can stimulate presynaptic alpha adrenergic receptor resulting in induction of a feed back mechanism which leads to inhibition of release of noradrenaline.

Major families of receptors based on transduction of a signal into a functional response

(a) **Receptors with intrinsic ion channels.** These are located on the cell surface. They enclose ion selective channels for Na^+, K^+, Ca^+, Cl^-. When an agonist is bound to these receptors they convey their signals, e.g., nicotinic cholinergic receptors (N_M).

(b) **Enzymatic receptors.** These receptors are enzyme molecule themselves, e.g., tyrosine protein kinase, threonine protein kinase, guanyl cyclase, etc.

© **G-protein coupled receptors.** These are located on cell membrane. G-protein is a connecting link between receptor and effector systems, like enzymes, carrier molecules, ion channels, etc. They are called G-proteins because of their link, with guanine nucleotides–GDP (guanosine diphosphate) and GTP (guanosine triphosphate). Two types of G-proteins are universally accepted: Gs (stimulatory type) and G_1 (inhibitory type). These receptors produce their pharmacological response through three major pathways:

• Adenyl cyclase /cAMP pathway (e.g. generation of cardiac impulse)

• Phospholipase C/ IP3 (inositol, 1,4,5 – triphosphate) – DAG (diacylglycerol) pathway (e.g. various types of secretary processes).

• Direct regulation of ion channels (e.g. muscarinic acetylcholine receptor present in heart muscle).

(d) **Intracellular receptors.** These are present either in cytoplasm or nucleus of the cell. Important drugs which act through such type of receptors are vitamin A, corticosteroids, vitamin D, etc.

Regulation of receptors

When receptors are exposed to an agonist for a long period of time, there is decrease in number of receptors or there may be diminished sensitivity. This is called *'desensitization'* phenomenon or down regulation of receptors. For example, levodopa when used for a long period slows down regulation of DA receptor (domaine) and naturally antiparkinsonian effect of levodopa is gradually lost. Similarly, when receptors are exposed to an antagonist for prolonged periods there is increase in number of receptors or increased sensitivity. This is called *supersensitivity or up-regulation of receptors*. For example, if timolol eye drop is stopped suddenly after prolonged use, there is every possibility of getting an acute attack of raised intra-ocular pressure.

Dose-Response Curve

When a drug is administered, it produces a response and this response shows alteration with the change in dose. The changes can be plotted with dose as abscissa and response as ordinate. The resulting curve is known as *dose-response curve*. Normally, after an initial phase, a time comes when increase in dose does not produce any increase in response. However, some drugs like loop diuretics produce responses with increase in dose for a longer period of time. Hence, these are called high ceiling diuretics.

Pharmacologically the response of a drug is determined by its molar concentration in tissues. There are two terms used in this regard: (i) graded response and (ii) quantal response.

Graded response. In this case, the dose-response curve rises steeply at first, but after that it becomes steady as the dose is increased. This type of curve is popularly known as *hyperbolic* or *exponential curve*. Such a curve can be shown by plotting dose against percent response. But if log dose is plotted against percent response, the curve obtained is a linear curve (Fig. 4.1 a)

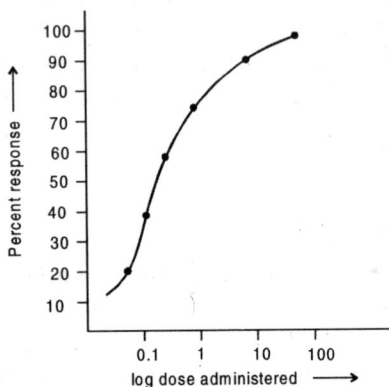

Fig. 4.1 a. Graded response curve

Quantal response. Here initially there is no appreciable response until a particular threshold is attained. Thereafter, the curve rises steeply until a maximum response is attained, but after this there is no appreciable change in the curve even with increased dose. This is called sigmoid or 'S' shaped curve and can be shown if log dose is plotted against percent data.

From the clinical point of view, there is no use of increasing dose of a drug which produces flat or shallow dose response curve (DRC). Therefore, a careful handling of a drug (regarding its dose), which shows steep DRC, is required.

A term called *drug potency* is often used to indicate the amount of drug required to produce a specific response. In case of lower potency drugs, the DRC is shifted rightwards. Another term called *efficacy* is used to denote the maximum amount of response which can be produced by the drug. The upper limit of DRC represents the efficacy of a drug. For example, aspirin in terms of its analgesic property is less potent and less efficacious than morphine (Fig. 4.1b).

Therapeutic Index

Therapeutic index is a measure of the relative safety of a drug for a particular treatment. It is the ratio between the toxic dose and the

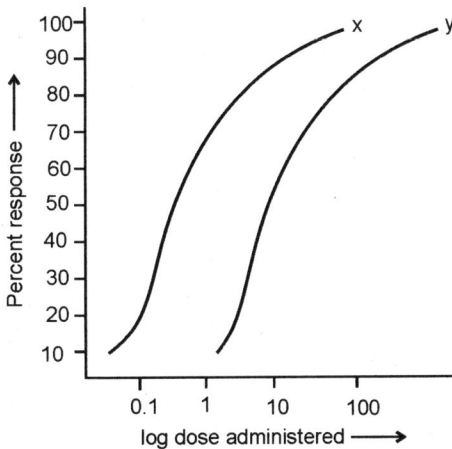

Fig. 4.1b. A diagram illustrating efficacy and potency in a log dose-response curve where log dose is plotted against response (Drug Y is less potent but is equally efficacious as drug X.)

therapeutic dose of a drug. In animal experiments, therapeutic index is calculated by the formula,

Therapeutic index = LD50/ED50,

Where LD 50 is the median lethal dose which can cause mortality in 50% of the animals which belong to same species and strain, and ED 50 is the median effective dose which can produce the required effect in 50% of the animals.

In clinical medicine, therapeutic index or margin of safety indicates the gap between the therapeutic effect DRC and adverse effect DRC.

Therapeutic Window Phenomenon

It is an interesting phenomenon observed with some drugs. Glipizide is an effective oral hypoglycaemic drug and the dose is 5 to 20 mg per day. But if the dose is increased to more than 25 mg/day, the glycaemia control power of the drug diminishes and such phenomenon is called therapeutic window phenomenon.

Various Terms Used in Relation to Drug Dosage

The term *dose* denotes appropriate amount of a drug required to produce a desired pharmacological action. A drug may produce different types of pharmacological effects depending on different types of dose. For example, anti-inflammatory dose of aspirin is 3 to 6 g per day, but platelet aggregation inhibitory dose is only 60 to 100 mg per day.

Loading dose means the dose required to achieve a target concentration rapidly. Thereafter, *maintenance dose* is used to retain the target level by balancing the elimination. Loading dose of doxycycline is 200 mg and the maintenance dose is 100 mg per day. Sometimes, a drug has to be adjusted by trial and error, viz., in open angle glaucoma first of all timolol (0.5%) BD is tried but if the desired level of IOP is not achieved, pilocarpine 2% BD is added to it. Such calculated doses are called *regulated doses*. There are some drugs like antineoplastic drugs whose dose is calculated by observing the onset of minimum level of appearance of toxic manifestations and such a drug dose is called *titrated dose*.

Factors Affecting the Action of a Drug

Following factors influence the pharmacological action of a drug:
- Factors related to the individual concerned.
- Genetic factors.
- Pharmacokinetic factors.
- Pathological status of body.
- Psychological and environmental factors.
- Drug-drug interaction with undesirable iatrogenic manifestations.
- Synergism and antagonism.
- Miscellaneous factors like tachyphylaxis, tolerance, cumulative action, resistance to drug, etc.

Factors Related to Individual Concerned

Age. In children, glomerular filtration rate is low and tubular secretion is subnormal. Hence, drugs like aminoglycoside antibiotics and penicillin should be used with caution in them. Similarly, in elderly people, drugs possessing anticholinergic activity may precipitate acute retention of urine as these individuals usually have some degree of prostatic enlargement.

Sex. Drugs like ketoconazole, beta blockers, etc., interfere with sexual activity in males. In females, established teratogenic drugs like corticosteroids should be avoided in second trimester of pregnancy. During pregnancy, the plasma albumin level decreases resulting in increase in free form of the acidic drugs and so the dose of NSAIDs should be adjusted accordingly.

Race. Incidence of aplastic anaemia due to chloramphenicol is less in Indians compared to the Anglo-Saxon race. Epidemic subacute myelo-optic neuropathy (SMON) following use of iodochloro-hydroxyquinoline has occurred in Japan, but such cases are practically unknown in India although consumption of the above drug is more in India.

Built. Dose may vary according to the size of the body. The most accurate way of dose calculation is on the basis of body surface area (BSA). The dose for children can be determined by utilizing this method.

Dose for the individual = {BSA (in m^2)/1.7} × average dose of the adult

According to Dubois formula, BSA (in m^2) = body weight (in kg) $^{0.425}$ × height (in cm)$^{0.725}$ × 0.007184.

Genetic Factors

An important example is precipitation of acute angle closure glaucoma on instillation of local mydriatic eye drop in genetically determined anatomically narrow irido-corneal angle individuals.

Pharmacokinetic Factors

Change of route of administration of a drug may alter the response of the drug in some cases. For example, glycerol when applied to dry skin surface softens it due to its emollient and demulcent property, but when taken internally by oral route it reduces intra ocular tension.

Pathological Status of the Body

In hepatic diseases as the serum albumin is reduced, free level of acidic drugs like NSAIDs, alprazolam, etc., may increase and so their dose should the adjusted. Drugs like acyclovir, vancomycin, etc., are totally contraindicated even in low degree renal failure cases.

In benign hyperplasia of prostate, administration of atropine eye drop topically for a long time may cause retention of urine.

Psychological and Environmental Factors

If a patient believes his physician and has full confidence in him, then even an inert substance (distilled water injection, lactose tablet, etc.) can induce remarkable analgesia. This effect is *placebo effect*. Placebo in Latin means *I shall please*. Recent evidences show that placebo substances release endorphins (endogenous opioid peptides) in brain, which have a powerful analgesic effect. The most important endorphin is beta endorphin (contains 31 amino acids) which is derived from pro-opio-melanocortin (POMC) and it acts mainly as an opioid receptor agonist. However, placebo effect is unreliable and shows many types of variations even in the same individual.

Environmental factors are also very important with regard to the action of a drug. For example, hypnotics act more perfectly in a suitable environment, particularly during night. Similarly, corticosteroids are given in the morning after breakfast to prevent pituitary adrenal suppression. A branch in pharmacology, called chronopharmacology, is coming up which deals with diurnal variation of human body and suitable time of drug administration to achieve a completely desirable response of a drug.

Drug-Drug Interactions with Undesirable Iatrogenic Factors

Timolol eye drop blocks both beta-1 and beta-2 adrenoreceptors and so in bronchial asthma patients, salbutamol fails to produce bronchodilatation and such condition may even be fatal. Similarly, aspirin, if used in a patient who is on spironolactone, may block the action of the latter by inhibiting the tubular secretion of canrenone (an important active metabolite of spironolactone).

Synergism and Antagonism

When two drugs are used together and the action of one drug is found to be increased by the other, the phenomenon is called synergism. In additive type of synergism, the effect perceived after administration of two drugs is not more than the sum of their individual actions, e.g., nitrous oxide and ether as general anaesthetics. But when such effect is found to be more than the sum of their individual actions, the type of synergism is called supradditive or potentiation, e.g., acetylcholine and physostigmine.

When two drugs are administered together and the effect perceived after administration is less than the sum of their individual actions, the phenomenon is called antagonism. Antagonism may be physio-chemical (e.g. chelation of iron by desferrioxamine), physiological (e.g. insulin and glucagons on blood sugar level), and receptor oriented (e.g. atropine antagonizes acetylcholine by blocking muscarinc receptors).

Miscellaneous factors

(a) **Tachyphylaxis**. It is a phenomenon seen in the case of indirectly acting drugs like ephedrine, tyramine, amphetamine, etc. Such drugs on repeated administration exhibit progressive decrease in vasopressor response. Even on increasing the dose, the effect is not observed. These drugs act by depletion of nor-adrenaline from sympathetic nerve endings. After repeated stimulation, the nor-adrenaline store gets totally exhausted and so the pharmacological action of drugs also stops. Now, if some time is allowed to lapse so that synthesis and accumulation of nor-adrenaline can take place, once again the indirectly acting drugs will produce the original pharmacological action in the same dose which was used initially. This phenomenon is called *tachyphylaxis.* Two more suggested factors concerned with tachyphylaxis are slow dissociation of drug molecule from the concerned receptor and diminution in number of receptors due to repeated stimulation.

(b) Tolerance. A drug on continuous use fails to give a particular response unless and until the dose is increased. Tolerance to a drug develops against a particular response and not to all responses. For example, morphine addict develops tolerance against euphoric and analgesic response but never against miosis and constipation effect.

Tolerance may be natural, e.g., African races show tolerance against mydriatics. It may be acquired, e.g., gradual increase in the dose of alcohol consumption in chronic alcoholics to get the desired euphoric effect. *Cross tolerance* means development of tolerance between two pharmacologically related but structurally different drugs, e.g., alcoholics show tolerance against general anaesthetics. *Pseudotolerance* or apparent tolerance means intentional development of tolerance, mainly against a poison like arsenic, by gradually and regularly consuming it in low dose, usually by oral route. But if the same poison is introduced in the system by any other route (e.g. I.M. injection), the tolerance developed by oral route fails to protect the person. Such type of tolerance is called pseudotolerance.

There are two main views regarding the cause of development of tolerance. One view suggests that on regular use, the drug molecules are quickly eliminated from the body and adequate receptor concentration is not achieved. This is called *pharmacokinetic tolerance.* The other view suggests that the drug receptors on chronic exposure lose affinity for that particular drug molecule. This is called *pharmacodynamic tolerance.* Whatever may be the cause, tolerance to a drug creates problem while treating a patient with a drug for a longer period of time.

(c) Cumulative action. A drug which is excreted slowly from the system, on continuous administration, may accumulate in toxic amount. This is called cumulative action, e.g., chloroquine on prolonged administration may cause retinal damage.

(d) Resistance against antimicrobial drugs. Microbes on chronic exposure to a drug often become apathetic to it and the drug loses its power to inhibit them. This phenomenon is called *drug resistance.* It may be natural, e.g., mycobacterium tuberculosis is inherently resistant to tetracyclines. It may be acquired, e.g., Staphylococcus aureus gets resistant to many antimicrobial agents. Such type of drug resistance develops either by mutation (single step or multistep) or by gene transfer (by conjugation or transduction or transformation).

Gene-Based Therapy

Gene-based therapy can produce a newer function. The basic idea behind such therapy is to replace a defective gene by a normal gene to control various inherited disorders and defects. In addition, such a therapy is also helpful in the management of various immunological diseases, malignancies and viral diseases like HIV.

Gene based therapy can be done by gene modification method, which is not so popular. In this method a defective gene can be removed and replaced by a new healthy gene or alternatively an extra gene can be introduced without removing the older defective one.

The more popular method is gene transfer method. In this method gene transfer can be done by liposomal delivery system or viral vector delivery system, the latter being more powerful. Viruses used are Herpes simplex, Adenovirus, Lentivirus, but the most effective are Retroviruses.

A recent advancement in gene therapy is introduction of antisense oligonucleotides, which can block the expression of a particular defective gene. Fomivirsen is such a compound, which has been approved for use in the management of CMV retinitis.

Adverse Drug Reactions (ADR)

According to WHO, ADR means "any response to a drug that is noxious and unintended and that occurs at doses used in man for prophylaxis, diagnosis or therapy". ADR can be divided into the following groups:

1. Side effects
2. Untoward reactions
3. Toxic manifestations
4. Drug intolerance
    (a) Quantitative intolerance
    (b) Qualitative intolerance
        (i) Idiosyncrasy
        (ii) Drug allergy
5. Organ toxicity related to drug therapy
    (a) Ocular
    (b) Non-ocular
6. Special Adverse drug reactions:
    (a) Carcinogenicity and mutagenicity
    (b) Teratogenicity
    (c) Drug dependence and withdrawal phenomenon
    (d) Iatrogenic disorders

1. Side Effects

A drug may possess many pharmacological actions. A particular drug is used to cure a particular clinical condition but other manifestations of that drug produced by therapeutic dose are termed as side effects. For example, in acute spasmodic condition of intestine, atropine injection is often prescribed. In some instances, the patient may develop an acute congestive attack of glaucoma due to anatomically narrow angle of anterior chamber, which is dangerous and undesirable. This happens due to mydriatic side effect of atropine causing crowding of angle by iris tissue. But in some instances, side effect of atropine may also be advantageous. For example, atropine used for pre-anaesthetic medication to prevent reflex inhibition of heart has a side effect called drying effect, which is advantageous for the patient undergoing general anaesthesia as there will be reduced bronchial secretion.

2. Untoward Reactions

These effects may occur even with therapeutic dose of a drug. For example, ethambutol, a widely used antitubercular drug, may cause dimness of vision, distorted colour vision, field changes, etc., due to optic neuritis. But if the medicine is stopped immediately the visual changes are reversible to a large extent.

3. Toxic Manifestations

These are more serious in nature and are usually seen in cases where a drug is consumed in high doses or when used for a prolonged period. For example, acetazolamide, when used for prolonged periods, may produce crystalluria and renal damage.

4. Drug Intolerance

When a person is unable to tolerate a drug even in therapeutic dose, the condition is called *drug intolerance*. For example, a single therapeutic dose of quinine may precipitate cinchonism. Drug intolerance may be quantitative or qualitative.

    A. Quantitative intolerance. There are some individuals who show hyper-reaction phenomenon even to sub-therapeutic dose of a drug. For example, a single dose of streptomycin injection may cause severe vertigo in susceptible individuals. This is known as quantitative intolerance.

    B. Qualitative intolerance. It is of two types : (i) idiosyncrasy and (ii) drug allergy

(i) Idiosyncrasy: In this type of reaction immune mechanisms do not play any role. In some individuals genetical deficiency or distortion or absence of an enzyme system has been observed. As for example, in people with glucose-6-phosphate dehydrogenase deficiency in RBC drugs like primaquine, sulfonamides, etc., produce haemolysis. Similarly in people with atypical type of plasma pseudocholinesterase, use of succinyl choline may cause respiratory palsy. But in some cases no such genetical problem can be demonstrated. As for example, idiosyncratic chloramphenicol induced agranulocytosis has no demonstrable genetical background.

(ii) *Drug allergy*: It is different from idiosyncrasy. It has got a positive immunological background and desensitization technique is applicable to many such drugs. In case of drug allergy, when a drug molecule enters in a susceptible individual, it acts like an antigen or combines with the body protein to form 'hapten', which in turn stimulates the immune system to form a specific antibody. This is the sequence that happens after first dose of the drug. When next dose is given, there is violent antigen-antibody reaction and in some cases such reaction may be fatal. Drug allergy or hypersensitivity can be categorized into two groups:

- *Humoral*: It includes anaphylactic reaction (Type I); cytolytic reaction (Type II) and immune complex mediated reaction (Arthus reaction, serum sickness) (Type III).
- *Cell mediated*: It includes delayed hypersensitivity reaction (Type IV).

Some pharmacologists also include Type V (anti-receptor type) reaction and Type VI (antibody dependent cell mediated cytotoxicity– ADCC). These two reactions are not included in the original classification of Gell and Coombs.

Management of drug allergy

The most dangerous, life threatening phenomenon of drug allergy is anaphylactic shock. The suggested line of management is as follows:

(i) The challenging allergen (drug) should be stopped immediately.

(ii) To combat edema larynx, adrenaline 0.5 mg. (0.5 ml. of 1 in 1000 solution) should be injected intramuscularly as quickly as possible; the dose may be repeated in obstinate cases after 5 to 10 min.

In addition to this oxygen therapy should be started urgently.

(iii) After adrenaline therapy, intravenous glucocorticoid (hydrocortisone sodium succinate -100 to 200 mg I.V. should be started. Adrenaline counteracts the effect of histamine (physiological antagonist) and glucocorticoids modify the immune mechanisms.

(iv) The role of combined H^1 and H^2 blockers for fully counteracting the role of histamine is also important.

For types II to VI the only effective treatment is corticosteroids.

Role of skin test for prevention of anaphylactic reaction

The best and most typical example is penicillin induced anaphylactic shock, which may be fatal. To prevent this, intradermal test with 2 to 10U of Penicillin is commonly done but this small amount may also cause anaphylactic shock. Now-a-days, this skin test is carried out by benzylpenicilloylpolylysine which is relatively safer. However, problem with such skin test is false positive or negative result. In some cases of negative skin test, delayed hypersensitivity phenomenon has been found to occur.

5. Organ Toxicity Related to Drug Therapy

Ocular

Many drugs may produce ocular toxicities. Adverse reactions of some important and commonly used drugs are as follows:

*   Hyperbaric oxygen therapy in premature infants may cause retrolental fibroplasia.
*   Corticosteroids may produce cataract, glaucoma, pseudotumour cerebri, etc.
*   Chloropromazine may produce cataract, retinopathy and light brown pigmentary changes in conjunctiva.
*   Prolonged chloroquine therapy may cause Bull's eye maculopathy, corneal changes and myopathy.
*   Indomethacin may produce corneal opacities.
*   Colour vision can be affected by drugs like ethambutol, digoxin, trimethadione, etc.
*   Sulphonamide derivatives like acetazolamide may cause Stevens-Johnson's syndrome.
*   Benign intracranial hypertension induced papilledema may be caused by hypervitaminosis A and oral contraceptives (in selective cases).
*   Quinine may destroy vision by inducing quinine amblyopia.
*   Rifampicin may produce orange coloured tears.

Non-ocular

Following drugs may produce toxicities in various organs:

*   Paracetamol overdose may cause liver cell necrosis by one of its metabolites called NABQI (N-acetyl-p-benzoquinoneimine).

- Chlorpromazine, erythromycin may cause cholestatic Jaundice.
- Isoniazide may produce hepatitis resembling viral hepatitis.
- Aminoglycoside antibiotics are nephrotoxic drugs.
- Chloramphenicol may produce agranulocytosis.
- d-Penicillamine may cause loss of taste sensation.
- Topical neomycin may cause contact dermatitis.
- Hydrallazine may produce SLE like lesions.
- Thiazide diuretics may cause gout and diabetes mellitus.
- Morphine may precipitate bronchial asthma.
- INH may cause peripheral neuritis.
- Reserpine may produce depressive psychosis.

6. Special Adverse Drug Reactions

(a) Carcinogenicity and mutagenicity

There are many drugs which may cause mutation of genes and on prolonged use may even cause cancer. The mechanisms by which such drugs act as carcinogens are very complex and discussion on this topic is beyond the scope of this book. One popular theory postulates generation of oxidative free radicals as a result of metabolic reactive processes. These free radicals (obtained from drug molecule) have unpaired electrons and, hence, they are highly reactive and are capable of damaging DNA molecule through a series of chain reactions. Drugs capable of producing mutagenesis include metronidazole, sodium cyclamate (a sweetening agent), radioactive isotopes, estrogens, etc.

Mutagenic potential of a drug can be studied by Ames Test. Normally, Salmonella typhimurium cannot thrive in a histidine-deficient medium. Now if the drug under investigation is mixed in such a medium and Salmonella typhimurium is found to grow (in histidine-deficient medium), the drug is believed to possess mutagenic potential.

(b) Teratogenicity

The greatest teratogenic tragedy which shook world was thalidomide tragedy (1958-61), which happened in Germany. Thalidomide was claimed to be a non-toxic hypnosedative and many pregnant women consumed it which resulted in about 2000 births with babies having seal-like limbs – the so called *phocomelia*. After this tragedy, human biologists focused their attention on teratogenic potentiality of drugs. Some drugs which act from conception to 17 days may interfere with continuation of pregnancy but it is very difficult to identify such drugs. A next set of drugs may affect the baby from 18th to 56th day which is the vital period of organogenesis. Such drugs may produce congenital deformities. A large set of drugs may affect fetus from 56th days onwards and this group may affect growth of internal organs (e.g. ACE inhibitors may cause hypoplasia of lung and kidneys) or may cause functional defect. Common drugs used in ophthalmology possessing teratogenic potentials are corticosteroids, atropine, aspirin, etc.

(c) Drug dependence and withdrawal syndrome

According to WHO, the drug dependence is defined as follows:

"A state, psychic and sometimes also physical, resulting from the interaction between a living organism and a drug, characterized by behavioural and other responses that always include a compulsion to take the drug on a continuous or periodic basis in order to experience its psychic effects and sometimes to avoid the discomfort of its absence. Tolerance may or may not be present. A patient may be dependant on more than one drug."

Psychic dependence means, craving to procure a drug at any cost and to consume it. Physical dependence means, if a drug is withdrawn there is withdrawal syndrome (because the system gets totally adaptive to the drug), which may be very mild or extremely violent (may be even fatal). Previously, a term was commonly used as *drug addiction*, which has recently been replaced by the term *drug abuse*. It means a compulsive desire to procure and consume the drug. Gradual increase in its dose and sudden abstention precipitates acute withdrawal syndrome. Pharmacologists believe that there is some sort of abnormal alteration in cellular metabolism of CNS, which is mainly responsible for drug dependence and abstinence causes acute withdrawal syndrome.

Common drugs capable of producing drug dependence are alcohol, hypnotics, opiates, amphetamine, cocaine, LSD, cannabis, tobacco, coffee, tea, etc. Treatment of drug dependence is very difficult but not impossible. Important therapies which help in treating such drug dependence cases include substitution therapy, psychotherapy, occupational therapy and lastly mass communication therapy cum rehabilitation therapy.

(d) Iatrogenic disorders

It means physician induced diseases. Some common examples of ophthalmological interest are as follows:

- Glucocorticoids may cause hypertension and diabetes mellitus on prolonged use.
- Timolol eye drop may precipitate fatal attack of bronchial asthma in asthmatic subjects.
- Chloramphenical eye drop may cause agranulocytosis.
- Acetazolamide may cause Stevens Johnson's syndrome.
- Atropine injection may precipitate an acute attack of glaucoma in individuals with anatomically narrow angle of anterior chamber.

CHAPTER 5

Antibacterials

Antibacterials are the substances or drugs that act against invading microorganisms known as "bacteria". Previously, they used to be synthesized from other microorganisms and were, therefore, named 'antibiotics'. Now, most of the antibacterials are produced synthetically from chemicals.

Basic Mechanisms of Action of Common Antibacterials

Following are the basic mechanisms of action of antibacterials.
1. By increasing cell membrane permeability causing leakage of cell material, e.g., polymyxins, bacitracin, etc.
2. By causing lysis of cell wall, e.g., penicillins, vancomycin, etc.
3. By suppressing the protein synthesis of bacteria, e.g., tetracycline, chloroamphenicol, erythromycin, clindamycin, etc.
4. By interfering with DNA function of bacteria, e.g., rifampicin, metronidazole.
5. By inhibiting DNA gyrase activity, e.g., fluoroquinolones.
6. By causing confusion of mRNA code and changing the permeability of bacteria, e.g., aminoglycosides.
7. By interfering in bacterial metabolism, e.g., sulfonamides, pyrimethamine, ethambutol, etc.

Some Important Drug Reactions with Antibiotics

- Jarisch-Herxheimer reaction—This is usually seen when penicillin is injected to syphilitic patients (particularly secondary syphilis) due to sudden release of body products of spirochetes (due to their lysis).

- Stevens-Johnson syndrome–It is associated with sulfonamides.

Common Toxicities of Some Important Antibiotics

- Chloramphenicol–bone marrow depression.
- Aminoglycosides–renal and 8th cranial nerve damage.
- Vancomycin–renal and ototoxicity.
- Polymyxin B–renal and neurological toxicity.
- Tetracyclines–hepatic and renal damage.
- Amphotericin B–bone marrow depression, neurological complications and renal damage.

Mechanisms of Development of Drug Resistance

There are two important processes by which a microbe may acquire resistance to a particular drug:

- Mutation, which may be single step or multi-step.
- Transfer of gene, which involves processes like conjugation, transformation and transduction.

By these mechanisms micro organisms get resistance by:

(1) Generation of a new metabolic pathway that does not involve the antimicrobial concerned.

(2) Development of new enzymes which break up the antimicrobial molecule.

(3) Alteration in membrane permeability so that effective concentration of the drug does not reach inside the microbial cell.

Concept of Cross Resistance

When an organism becomes resistant to a particular drug it also exhibits resistance towards some other drugs which are usually structurally (chemical) related to that drug. Example: resistance developed to a particular sulfonamide means resistance to whole group. This is called *cross-resistance*. However, there are some exceptions to this law, e.g., patients resistant to gentamycin (an aminoglycoside) may respond to amikacin (another aminoglycoside).

Cross-resistance is of two types:
(a) *Two way cross-resistance*: Resistance to erythromycin means usually resistance to clindamycin and vice versa.
(b) *One way cross-resistance*: Resistance to neomycin usually means resistance to streptomycin also, but those resistant to streptomycin may respond to neomycin.

Therapeutic guidelines to avoid resistance problem

The therapeutic guidelines to avoid microbial resistance are:
(1) When prolonged drug therapy is decided (e.g. tubercular infection), multiple drugs should be started at a time.
(2) When the treatment is for a microbe of high pathogenicity (e.g. *E. coli*), drug therapy should be continued till the microbes are totally eradicated.
(3) When the treatment is for a microbe of low pathogenicity, unnecessary lengthy period of treatment should be avoided. Care should also be taken in the selection of drug. It should be specific (narrow spectrum).

Antibiotics to be avoided during pregnancy

Aminoglycosides, chloramphenicol, tetracycline, fluoroquinolones, sulfonamides, nitrofurantoin, etc., should be avoided in pregnancy because they either have teratogenic effect or may deteriorate fetomaternal well being.

Superinfection

Super infection means development of a new infection while using antimicrobial agents. This is due to the destruction of normal bacterial flora. Normal flora serves two defensive functions: it (1) liberates a chemical called bacteriocin, which inhibits pathogens, and (2) it deprives the pathogens from nutrients, i.e., pathogens have to compete with normal flora for nutrition.

Super infection usually occurs more easily in patient suffering from AIDS, diabetes mellitus, bone-marrow depression, and patients undergoing chemotherapy (for malignant diseases), prolonged use of immunosuppressive and corticosteroids, etc.

The causative organisms usually responsible for super infection are: Staphylococci, Candida albicans, proteus group, pseudomonas group, Clostridium difficile, etc.

To avoid super infection, antimicrobials should not be used indiscriminately (example: prolonged antibiotic therapy in simple virus infections).

Rationale for Polytherapy

Multiple antimicrobial therapy is justified in the following circumstances:
- When causative organisms may be multiple and the health condition of the patient is poor.
- To get additive effect, e.g., Sulfonamide + Trimethoprim.
- To reduce toxic reactions, to avoid superinfection and to reduce the chances of production of drug resistance.

Risks of Polytherapy

- Production of resistant strain if proper combination is not used.
- Drug toxicity may be enhanced, e.g., while using vancomycin with tobramycin.
- There may be more severe type of superinfection.
  In third world countries cost of therapy should also be considered.

Prophylactic Antimicrobial Therapy

The role of prophylactic antimicrobial therapy is controversial. However, in some circumstances it may be justified as follows:
- Patients undergoing surgery, dental extraction, endoscopies, etc.
- Road accidents.
- Children or people with low immunity when residing with open tuberculosis cases.
- In situations like exposure to malaria (in endemic areas), meningococcal meningitis (during an epidemic), syphilis and gonorrhoea (immediately before or after contact) prophylactic antimicrobial therapy is justified.

Specific Antimicrobial Agents

Important classes of antibacterial agents are:
(1) Sulfonamides
(2) Co-trimoxazole, Pyrimethamine
(3) Quinolones
(4) Antibiotics:
   (a) Beta lactam antibiotics, e.g., Penicillins, Cephalosporins, Monobactams and Carbapenems.
   (b) Broad spectrum antibiotics, e.g., Tetracyclines and Chloramphenicol.
   (c) Aminoglycoside antibiotics, e.g., Streptomycin, Gentamycin, Tobramycin, Amikacin, Sisomicin, Netilmicin, Framycetin, etc.
   (d) Macrolide antibiotics, e.g., Erythromycin, Roxithromycin, Clarithromycin, Azithromycin.
(5) Miscellaneous agents: Clindamycin, Vancomycin, Teicoplanin, Fusidic acid, Mupirocin, Spectinomycin, Polypeptide antibiotics, Metronidazole, Antiseptics and some recently developed drugs.

Sulfonamides

Mechanism of action

Sulfonamides are bacteriostatic agents. These agents cause competitive inhibition of bacterial folate synthetase, an enzyme needed for incorporation of p-aminobenzoic acid (PABA) into folic acid, a vital compound needed for bacterial growth. Besides, it is also believed that sulfonamides, due to their structural similarly to PABA (Fig.5.1), are taken up by mistake (by the bacteria) and there is formation of altered folate which is metabolically injurious to the organism concerned.

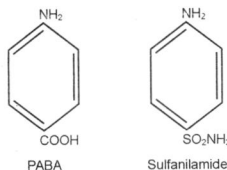

Fig. 5.1. Chemical structures of PABA and sulfanilamide

Co-trimoxazole

The combination of sulfamethoxazole (400 mg) and trimethoprim (80 mg) in the ratio of 5:1 is called co-trimoxazole when combined as a single unit. It acts as a bacteriocidal agent.

Mechanism of action

As already stated, sulfonamides inhibit the enzyme dihydropteroate synthetase and prevent the formation of dihydropteroic acid which is an immediate precursor of folic acid. Trimethoprim inhibits the enzyme dihydrofolate reductase so that tetrahydrofolic acid cannot be formed. This phenomenon is called sequential blockade of folate mechanism. It is interesting to note that both individual components of co-trimoxazole are bacteriostatic, but as a unit it acts as bactericidal agent. Since purulent exudates contain a large amount of PABA, the effect of sulfonamide is hampered to some extent under such situations.

Ophthalmic uses

(1) Topically sulfacetamides (solution 30% or ointment 10%) are used in corneal infections, conjunctival infections, etc.

(2) Initial treatment of toxoplasmosis is done by combination of sulfadiazine and pyrimethamine (given for 4 to 6 weeks). More obstinate cases are treated with co-trimoxazole, prednisolone and clindamycin.

(3) In nocardial keratitis, a topical broad spectrum antibiotic along with systemic co-trimoxazole therapy brings quick resolution.

(4) In trachoma and inclusion conjunctivitis, topical sulfacetamide sodium (10% to 30% × 4 weeks) along with systemic tetracycline therapy gives beneficial results.

(5) In burn cases involving eye lid, topical silver sulfadiazine or mafenide gives good protection against infection.

Side effects

Adverse reactions to sulfonamides are common. These may be:

1. Features of G.I. tract irritation like nausea, vomiting, anorexia, epigastric discomfort, etc.

2. Renal toxicities including crystalluria, haematuria, etc. However, plenty of fluid administration and alkalinization of

urine (alkaline urine makes sulfonamides and their derivatives more soluble) reduces this problem.

3. Hypersensitive type of hepatitis is sometimes seen (0.1%).
4. Many other types of hypersensitive reactions may occur (viz. drug fever, urticaria, polyarteritis nodosa, arthritis, etc.), but the most dangerous is Stevens-Johnson syndrome.
5. In individuals with G-6-PD deficiency, haemolysis may occur. In some individuals bone-marrow depression also occurs.
6. Precipitation of kernicterus may occur in premature infants due to displacement of bilirubin from plasma albumin.
7. Transient myopia (due to ciliary edema), toxic amblyopia, formation of white plaque (crystals of sulfonamide), etc., have been reported.

Drug interactions

1. Sulfonamides enhance the action of warfarin, tolbutamide, phenytoin, etc., by inhibiting their metabolism and by displacing them from their protein binding sites.
2. Sulfonamides may increase the chances of toxicity of methotrexate by displacing it from its binding site and by depressing its renal excretion.
3. Sulfonamides may counteract the efficiency of gentamycin (particularly, when it is used to treat pseudomonas infection).

Quinolones

Quinolones are synthetic chemical compounds. The parent compound is nalidixic acid (Fig.5.2). It is a weak antimicrobial substance. Some

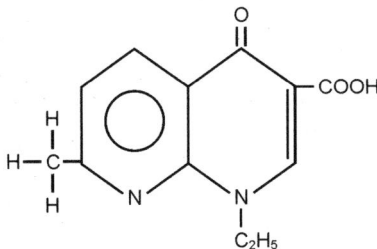

Fig. 5. 2. Chemical structure of nalidixic acid

newer quinolone substances, fluoroquinolones, have been developed by introducing one or more fluorine substituents. These are powerful antimicrobial substances.

Classification of fluoroquinolones

Fluoroquinolones are classified into two categories: first and second generation fluoroquinolones. The first generation drugs have one fluoro substitution, e.g., ciprofloxacin, norfloxacin (Fig. 5.3), ofloxacin, pefloxacin, etc. The second generation drugs have additional fluoro and other substituents. These drugs have extended spectrum of activity and are metabolically more stable. Examples: gatifloxacin, sparfloxacin, lomefloxacin, etc.

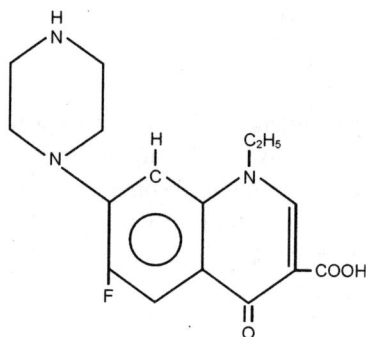

Fig. 5. 3. Chemical structure of norfloxacin

Spectrum of activity

- Quinolones (nalidixic acid) are mainly active against Gram-negative bacteria.
- 1st generation fluoroquionolones (prototype: ciprofloxacin): The most susceptible are aerobic Gram-negative organisms like enterobacteriaceae and Neisseria group. Gram positive organisms are susceptible at relatively higher concentration. Some organisms exhibit low or variable sensitivity, e.g., Mycoplasma, Chlamydia, Streptococcus faecalis, Streptococcus pneumoniae, Mycobacterium kansasii, Mycobacterium avium, etc. Organisms which are resistant include anaerobic cocci, clostridia group, Bacteroides fragilis, etc.

- 2nd generation fluoroquinolones, e.g., sparfloxacin exhibits more powerful action against Gram-positive organisms like enterococci, staphylococci, pneumococci, anaerobes, Mycobacterium tuberculosis, Mycobacterium avium, Mycobacterium leprae, etc.

Mechanism of action

All fluoroquinolones exhibit anti-DNA gyrase activity. While multiplying, the bacteria needs DNA gyrase for division, coiling and supercoiling of its DNA molecules.

- Topoisomerase II is the homologous enzyme in mammalian cell which has very low affinity for fluoroquinolones and so the toxicity to host cell is minimum. Resistant organisms detected show:
- Chromosomal mutation which produces a special type of DNA gyrase which has low affinity for fluoroquinolones. Permeability to the drug is reduced.

Ophthalmic use

Ciprofloxacin. In bacterial keratitis, it produces good response. Intravitreal injection is safe up to the dose 0.1 mg.
Topical use: 0.3% drop 4 times a day (in more acute cases even 1 hourly interval may be used.
Systemic use: 250 mg to 750 mg as tablets twice daily. I.V. infusion 200 mg 12 hourly is usually sufficient.

Norfloxacin. It is less powerful than ciprofloxacin. Topical use: 0.3% drops 4 times a day (even at one hourly intervals).
Systemic use: 400 mg tablets twice daily.

Ofloxacin. Its penetration into anterior chamber is better than that of ciprofloxacin and aminoglycosides;
0.3% eye drop is usually used.
Systemic use: The dose is 200 mg to 400 mg tablet daily.

Pefloxacin. It is used as 0.3% solution topically and 400 mg tablet twice daily systemically.

Lomefloxacin. It is also used topically 0.3% and systemically (400 mg. tablet once daily).

Sparfloxacin. It gives a higher aqueous and vitreous concentration compared to ciprofloxacin. Oral dose is 400 mg as a single loading dose followed by 200 mg per day.

Gatifloxacin. It is more effective than ciprofloxacin and *levofloxacin* is active against multiple drug resistant staphylococci. It is available as 0.3% solution. Usual oral dose is 400 mg per day.

Moxifloxacin. 0.5% eye drop is available for topical use and 400 mg tablet–once a day orally.

Adverse effects

- G.I. tract irritation – Nausea, vomiting, anorexia and, very rarely, pseudomembranous colitis.
- Nalidaxic acid may produce haemolytic anaemia in patients with G-6 phosphate dehydrogenase deficiency.
- A few cases of tendonitis have been reported.
- CNS reactions include headache, insomnia, confusion and, very rarely, convulsions.
- Hypersensitive reactions like photosensitivity, dry rash, swelling of lips, urticaria, etc.

Contraindications

Since fluoroquinolones may cause damage to the cartilage of juvenile weight bearing bones, so these should not be used in children. These should also be avoided in pregnancy and lactation.

Drug interactions

- Antacids reduce their absorption.
- H2 blockers reduce their absorption.
- There is increased susceptibility of convulsions when quinolones are used along with NSAID.
- Ciprofloxacin by reducing the metabolism of theophyllines may produce toxicity.
- Nalidaxic acid and nitrofurantoins are antagonistic.

Beta Lactam Antibiotics

1. Penicillins

Original Source: A fungus – Penicillium notatum; *present source* -- a high yielding mutant of Penicillium chrysogenum.

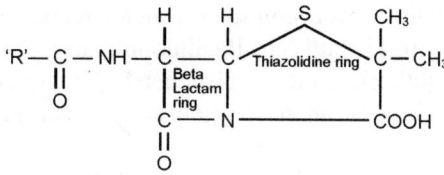

Fig. 5.4. Basic chemical structure of penicillins

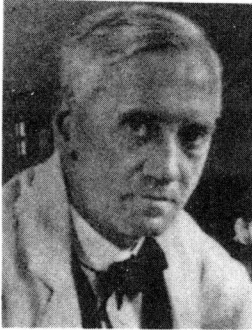

Fig.5.5. Sir Alexander Fleming – discoverer of penicillin

Penicillin nucleus consists of two rings – thiazolidine and beta lactam, which are fused together (Fig. 5.4). To this nucleus, side chains are attached by an amide linkage.

Mechanism of action

Beta lactam antibiotics cause damage to the bacterial cell wall. Hence, they are basically bacteriocidal agents. They (beta lactam) inhibit two important enzymes transpeptidase and carboxypeptidase, which are responsible for synthesis of peptidoglycan (a very important constituent of bacterial cell wall). As a result, rapid lysis of cell occurs. This lysis is augmented by activation of autolysins.

Classification

(1) *Classical penicillins*: These can be divided into two groups acid labile and acid resistant penicillins.

    (a)   Acid labile penicillins, e.g., Benzylpenicillin (penicillin G), Procaine penicillin G, Benzathine penicillin G -- These are active against Streptococci (except group D), pneumococci, gonococci, meningococci, many Gram-positive bacilli (viz. Bacillus anthracis, Corynebacterium diphtheriae, etc.), spirochetes (Treponema pallidum, etc.). These are moderately active against organisms like Actinomyces israelii.

Most of the Gram-negative bacilli, Mycobacterium group, Rickettsiae, fungus, chlamydae, viruses, protozoa, etc., are totally insensitive.

    (b) Acid resistant penicillin, e.g., Phenoxymethylpenicillin or Penicillin V – The spectrum of activity is more or less similar to that of benzyl penicillin but is less potent.

(2) *Penicillinase-resistant penicillins:*
These include cloxacillin, methicillin, nafcillin, oxacillin, etc. These are mainly active against penicillinase producing staphylococci.

(3) *Extended spectrum penicillins:*
    (a) Broad spectrum penicillins -- Ampicillin, amoxicillin, etc. These are also called amino-penicillins.

Spectrum includes (in addition to those sensitive to penicillin G) many Gram-negative bacilli like H influenzae, E. coli, Salmonella group, Shigella group, etc. Penicillinase producing staphylococci are not affected.

    (b) Antipseudomonal penicillins -- (i) Carboxy penicillins, e.g., ticarcillin, carbenicillin, etc., and (ii) Ureidopenicillins, e.g., piperacillin, mezlocillin, etc.

Carboxypenicillins are very much active against Pseudomonous aeruginosa and indole positive proteus, while Ureidopenicillins are active against Pseudomonas and Klebsiella.

(4) Special type penicillins ,e.g., Mecillinam, Temocillin:
These drugs produce lysis of bacterial cell wall in a different way than conventional penicillins. They are mainly active against aerobic Gram-negative enterobacilli (E coli, Klebsiella, Enterobacter, Salmonella, etc.). They have no action against Pseudomonas or Gram-positive cocci.

Beta lactamase inhibitors

Clavulanic acid, Sulbactam and Tazobactam are important members of this group. Clinically, these compounds are used along with penicillins to offer protection against beta-lactamase.

Important drug combinations available are:
Ampicillin + Sulbactam – I.V. or I.M.
Piperacillin + Tazobactam – I.M.
Ticarcillin + Clavulanic acid – I.V.
Amoxycillin + Clavulanic acid – oral.

Dosage

(a) Crystalline penicillin injection: 0.5 to 5 MU I.M. / I.V. every 6 to 12 hours.
(b) Procaine penicillin G injection: 0.5 to 1 MU I.M. every 12 to 24 hours.
(c) Benzathine penicillin G: 0.6 to 2.4 MU I.M. every 2 to 4 weeks.
(d) Penicillin V (phenoxymethyl penicillin): adults – 250-500 mg, 6 hourly; children – 125-250 mg, 6 hourly; infants – 60 mg, 6 hourly.
(e) Cloxacillin: 0.25 to 0.5 g. Orally – 6 hourly. In serious infections 0.25 to 1 g. I.M. or I.V.
(f) Ampicillin: adults – 0.5 to 2 g. Oral/I.M./I.V. depending upon seriousness of the condition, every 6 hours; children – 25-50 mg/kg/day.
(g) Amoxicillin: 0.25 to 1 g. Thrice daily orally.
(h) Carbenicillin: Na salt is used – 1 to 2 g. I.M. or 1 to 5 g. I.V. every 4 to 6 hours.
(i) Piperacillin: 100 to 150 mg/kg of the body wt. per day in three divided doses; total dose should not exceed 16 g/day – I.M./I.V.

Ocular penetration

Ocular penetration capacity of various penicillin compounds is poor; 0.5 to1 million units of penicillin G, given subconjunctivally produce effective therapeutic level in aqueous humour and vitreous. Its renal excretion can be slowed down by concurrent use of probenecid, 500 mg twice daily. Probenecid also retards the pumping effect of RPE (Retinal Pigment Epithelium) and thereby reduces elimination of penicillin from eye. Intraocular penetration of ampicillin is satisfactory.

Adverse effects

- Most important is penicillin shock (anaphylactic reaction). Other hypersensitive reactions of milder nature include serum sickness, drug rash, drug fever, bronchospasm, etc. Exfoliative dermatitis and Steven Johnson syndrome have also been reported.
- Oxacillin and nafcillin may occasionally cause bone marrow depression.
- Intrathecal injection is no more popular due to complications like encephalopathy, spinal cord damage, etc.
- Jarisch-Herxheimer reaction is seen in syphilitic cases.

Management of penicillin shock

- Corticosteroids, viz., hydrocortisone hemisuccinate – 100 mg I.V.
- Adrenaline – given subcutaneously 0.5 ml. to 1 ml.
- Oxygen therapy (in desperate cases tracheostomy, artificial respiration, etc.)
- I.V. fluid therapy.
- Aminophylline – I.V. – 250 mg
- Beta 2 agonists like salbutamol (0.25 to 0.5 mg. I.M. /S.C.) may be given.
- Antihistamines like chlorpheniramine (0.1 mg/kg I.M.)
- In case of pulmonary edema, furosemide – 40 mg. I.V. may be given.

Drug interactions

- Aminoglycosides should not be mixed with penicillins in the same drip.
- Anticoagulants + large I.V. dose of penicillin: chance of bleeding as bleeding time is prolonged.
- Oral contraceptives may lose potency if used with penicillins. So, an additional method of contraception should be adopted during this period.
- Parenteral penicillins plus heparin – there is increased chance of bleeding

- Allopurinol increases the allergic skin rash produced by ampicillin.
- Tetracycline (bacteriostatic) may hamper the bacteriocidal effect of penicillins.
- Probencid increases the half life of penicillins.

2. Cephalosporins

They are semi-synthetic antibiotics obtained from a fungus cephalosporium and they possess a beta lactam ring (Fig. 5.6). They are bactericidal in nature and cause damage to bacterial cell wall. However, their mechanism of action (as regards to protein binding) is a little different from that of penicillins.

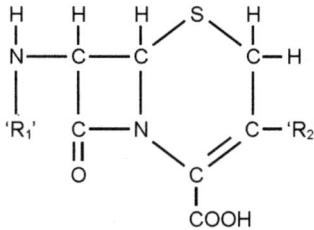

Fig. 5. 6. Basic chemical structure of cephalosporins

Classification

Cephalosporins are divided into four generations according to their time of entry into therapeutic field. But more important is their spectrum of activity and potency.

First generation. Introduced in 1960s, they are highly effective against Gram-positive cocci but are moderately effective against a few Gram-negative enterobacilli. Important members of this group are cefazolin, cephalexin, cephradin, cefadroxil, etc.

Second generation. Introduced between 1960 and 1980, they are more effective against Gram-negative organisms; some members of this group are effective against anaerobes (cefoxitin, cefotetan, cefmetazole). Important members of this group are cefuroxime, cefaclor, etc.

Third generation. Introduced in 1980s, they have powerful activity against Gram-negative enterobacteriaceae. Some compounds (cefoperazon, cefatazidime) are very effective against Pseudomonas. The powerful agents against Enterobacteriaceae are cefotaxime, ceftriaxone, ceftazidime, etc.

Fourth generation. They were introduced in 1990s; they have similar antibacterial spectrum as the third generation, but the compounds are highly resistant to beta lactamases. The important members are cefepime, cefpirome, etc.

Orally active compounds

1st generation – Cephalexin, cephradine, cephadroxil.
2nd generation – Cefuroxime axetil, Cefaclor.
3rd generation – cefixime.

Pharmakokinetics

Chephalospoins are absorbed in adequate amounts from oral routes, I.M./I.V. preparation: and quickly attain adequate blood concentration. They are basically excreted through renal route. Cephalosporins like cefotaxime are deacetylated in the body and their metabolites are also pharmacologically active agents. Cefoperazone is mainly eliminated through bile. Important cephalosporins which can cross blood-brain barrier are ceftizoxime, cefotaxime, cefuroxime and ceftriaxone and are useful in meningitis. All cephalosporins can appear in synovial fluid, aqueous humour, pericardial fluid and can cross placental barrier.

Dosage and preparation of some commonly used cephalosporins

1st generation:
    (a) Cefradroxil – 0.5 to 1 g, BD orally.
    (b) Cephazolin – 0.25 g, 8 hourly I.M. /I.V.; 1 g, 6 hourly I.M./ I.V. (severe cases)
    (c) Cephalexin – 0.25-1 g, 6 to 8 hourly (adults) 25 to 100 mg/ kg/day (children) all orally.
    (d) Cephadrine – 0.25 to 1 g, 6 to 12 hourly, oral / I.M./I.V.
2nd generation:
    (a) Cefuroxime axetil – 250-500 mg, BD (adults); 125-250 mg, BD (children)
    b) Cefoxitine – 1 to 2 g, every 6 to 8 hours I.M. /I.V.

3rd generation:
  (a) Cefixime – 200-400 mg, BD orally.
  (b) Ceftazidime – 0.5 to 2 g, 8 hourly I.M. /IV (adults); 30 mg/
     kg/day (children).
  (c) Cefoperazone – 1-2 g, 12 hourly I.M. /I.V. (adults); 50-100
     mg/kg/day (children).
4th generation:
  Cefpirome – 1-2 g, 12 hourly I.M. /I.V.

Intraocular penetration

Experiments have shown that intravitreal penetration of cephalosporins is not good. For example, a subconjunctival injection of ceftazidime or cefotaxime produces adequate concentration in vitreous cavity only in aphakic or vitrectomised eyes and not in normal eyes. So, ceftazidime is used (2.25 mg) as intravitreal injection in the management of bacterial endophthalmitis.

Adverse effects

  • Cephalosporins have cross sensitivity with penicillins and so
    only 10% of the patients who are hypersensitive to penicillin
    show equal response to cephalosporins. Therefore, it is wise
    to avoid cephalosporins in penicillin sensitive persons.
    Moreover, skin test with cephalosporin is unreliable.
  • Oral cephradine and parenteral cefoperazone may produce
    diarrhoea.
  • Some cephalosporins like cephalothin (having low grade
    nephrotoxicity), if used concurrently with aminoglycosides
    or loop diuretics, may cause renal toxicity, particularly in
    patients with depressed renal function.
  • Ceftazidime type of cephalosporins may produce neutropenia
    and thrombocytopenia.
  • Cefoperazone exhibits a disulfiram like action, if alcohol is
    ingested.
  • Cefoperazone and ceftriaxone may produce bleeding due to
    hypoprothrombinaemia, particularly in patient with renal
    failure.
  • Thrombophlebitis after I.V. injection is an important problem
    in the case of cephalosporins.

Drug Interactions

- Concurrent use of cephalosporins like cephalexin, cefazolin, etc., with aminoglycosides or furosemide may produce nephrotoxicity.
- Probenecid, by blocking the tubular secretion, prolongs the half life of drugs like cefadroxil, cefazoline, etc.
- Cephalosporins like cefadroxil, cefazolin, etc., potentiate the hypoprothrombinaemic effect of anticoagulants.
- Cephalosporins like cefoperazone, ceftriaxone, etc., may produce disulfiram like action with alcohol.
- Chloramphenicol antagonises the action of cephalosporins like ceftazidime.
- Cefazolin, cefadroxil, etc., produce false positive urinary glucose test. Direct Coomb's test and false elevated levels of urinary 17-ketosteroid values.

3. Monobactams

In this group of antibiotics only beta lactam ring is present and the second ring (characteristic of penicillins and cephalosporins) is missing. Aztreonam is the classical drug in this group.

Spectrum of activity

In low concentration, it inhibits Gram-negative enteric bacilli and *H. influenzae* and in moderately high concentration it may also inhibit Pseudomonas group. It is not inactivated by most of the beta lactamase.

It can be used in penicillin and cephalosporin hypersensitive cases, as there is no cross sensitivity of monobactams with them.

Dosage and preparation

0.5-2 g, 6 to 12 hourly I.M. /I.V.

4. Carbapenems

Imipenem is the most popular drug of this group. It is a very potent, beta lactamase-resistant, broad spectrum beta lactam antibiotic. It is active against Gram-positive cocci, Peudomonas group, anaerobes like *B. fragils* and *Cl. difficile*, enterobacteriacae, etc. It gets inactivated by an enzyme called dehydropeptidase I, situated on the brush border of renal tubular cells. To overcome this problem, a compound called cilastatin is used along with impenem which protects it by inhibiting (reversible) the enzyme dehydropeptidase I.

Dosage

Imipenem-cilastatin combination – 0.5 g, every 6 hours I.V. (not exceeding a dose of 4 g/ day).

Side effects

Usually milder side effects like nausea, vomiting are seen. Hypersensitive reactions may also occur (cross sensitivity is seen with other beta lactams). It may produce convulsions when high doses are used.

Ocular penetration

It penetrates well into the eye. Experiments have shown that following an I.V. injection of 1 g Imipenem, the minimal inhibitory concentration (MIC) for 90% of the susceptible bacteria is reached within a short period in the vitreous. So, it is a drug of choice in bacterial endophthalmitis.

Meropenem: It is also a carbapenem derivative and is not affected by renal dehydropeptidase I and is effective against Imipenem resistant Pseudomonas.

Broad Spectrum Antibiotics

Chloramphenicol

Originally derived from Streptomyces venezuelae, chloramphenicol (Fig. 5.7) is now totally synthetically produced for commercial purposes.

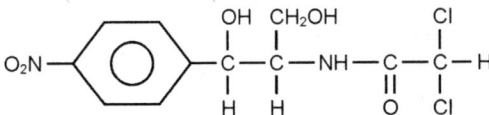

Fig. 5.7. Chemical structure of chloramphenicol

Mechanism of action

It is mainly bacteriostatic in nature, but is bactericidal in case of *H. influenzae*. It gets bound to 50S ribosomal subunit and thereby inhibits bacterial protein synthesis. Binding of aminoacyl-t RNA to 50S ribosomal subunit is prevented by it and thus peptide bond formation is ultimately hampered.

Spectrum of activity

A broad spectrum antibiotic, it is active against a wide range of organisms. Both Gram-positive and Gram-negative aerobic and anaerobic microorganisms as also chlamydiae, rickettsia and mycoplasma group of organisms are susceptible to this drug.

Choramphenicol in ophthalmology

Because of its wide spectrum and low propensity for generation of microbial resistance, it is the most popular topically used antibiotic. But its only risk is development of non-dose dependant bones marrow aplasia, which is usually fatal. However, most of the ophthalmologists use it with proper caution (family history and personal history of drug allergy) and for a small period. Even today about more than 90% of bacteria infecting conjunctiva and adenexa are susceptible to it. Although it is highly lipid soluble, its penetration is limited to cornea and aqueous humour. Adequate concentration is not achieved in vitreous.

Dosage

In ophthalmology, 0.4% to 0.5% solution (eye drop) and 1% eye ointment usually used for topical use.

Adverse effects

- The most dangerous complication is bone-marrow depression which may be dose-independent idiosyncratic reaction or dose-related depression.
- Others include G.I. tract irritation features, drug rash, drug fever, super infection, etc.
- Gray baby syndrome – It usually occurs in premature infants who receive high dose as prophylactic antiinfective therapy.

These children are unable to metabolize the drug due to lack of enzyme. As a result, a toxic manifestation like vomiting, anorexia, hypotonia, distended abdomen, appearance of ash colored grey cyanosis, followed by cardiovascular collapse, ending in death may occur. Lactic acid level also shoots up.

Drug Interactions

* Metabolism of certain drugs is inhibited by chloramphenicol. They are oral hypoglycaemics (chlorpropamide, tolbutamide), phenytoin sodium, cyclophosphamide, warfarin, etc.
* Certain drugs enhance the metabolic degradation of chloramphenicol so much so that failure of therapy may develop. These drugs are rifampicin, phenobarbitone, etc.

(Note: Phenytoin metabolism is inhibited by chloramphenicol, but phenytoin by inducing microsomal enzymes increases degradation of chloramphenicol).

Tetracyclines

Tetracyclines are a group of broad-spectrum antibiotics, effective against a wide variety of bacteria. The first drug of the tetracycline family, chlortetracycline was introduced in 1948. As the name implies, chemical structure of these antibiotics (Fig. 5.8) contains 4 cyclic rings. All members of this group are isolated from soil actinomycetes. As mentioned earlier, the first antibiotic of this group was chlortetracycline, which was isolated from Streptomyces aureofaciens.

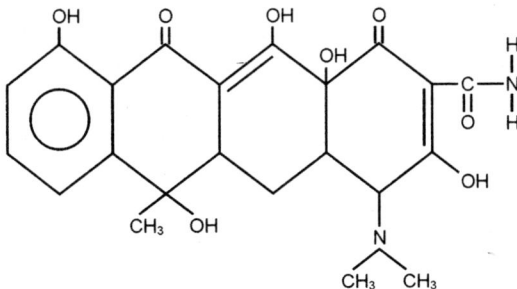

Fig. 5.8. Chemical structure of tetracycline

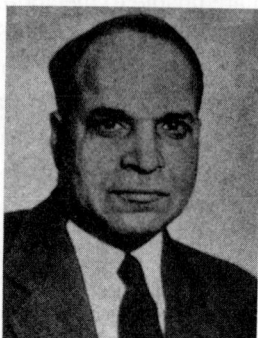

Fig. 5.9. Dr Subba Rao – discoverer of chlortetracycline along with Duggar

According to the chronology of their development, they are broadly divided in 3 groups:

Group 1: Tetracycline, oxytetracycline and chlortetracycline.
Group 2: Methacycline, demeclocycline, lymecycline.
Group 3: Minocycline, doxycycline.

Mechanism of action

Tetracyclines are bacteriostatic. They get bound to 30S ribosomes of the susceptible organism. And so attachment of aminocyl-t-RNA to m-RNA ribosome complex is hampered leading to failure of the development of peptide chain. Thus, the protein synthesis is inhibited.

Spectrum of activity

When introduced originally, tetracyclines were active against a wide variety of organisms, both Gram-positive and -negative cocci and bacilli, but today many organisms have acquired resistance against them. Mycobacterium tuberculosis, leprae are not susceptible. Other organisms worth mentioning are rickettsia, mycoplasma and chlamydia. Some protozoa, like amoeba, and plasmodium group are susceptible at high concentrations. The organisms which have become insensitive to tetracycline include staphylococci, pseudomonas and proteus group.

In ophthalmology the main indications of tetracycline include chlamydial infection (trachoma, inclusion blenorrhea of newborn), ulcerative blepharitis, rosacea, etc. Minocycline has proved to be effective against toxoplasmosis and phlyctenular conjunctivitis. As such, ocular penetration of tetracyclines is poor except for doxycycline and minocycline (which are found in 50% concentration of serum).

Mechanism of development of resistance

*   Bacteria acquire a special type of property for pumping out of tetracycline.
*   Concentration mechanism of tetracycline is less pronounced.
*   Bacteria produce a special protein which protects it from binding effect of the drug at the ribosomal binding site.

Preparation and dosage

*   Tetracycline oral: 1 g daily in 2 to 4 divided doses (adults can be given parenteraly also. 1% eye / ear drops and 3% skin ointment is also available).
*   Oxytetracycline: Adults (oral) 1 g/ day in 4 divided doses. Injection is also available (250 g once every 24 hr). 1% eye/ ear drops and 3% skin ointment is also available.
*   Chlortetracycline: Adults (oral) 1 g/ day in 2 to 4 divided doses. 1% eye ointment and 3% skin ointment is available.
*   Demeclocycline: Adults 600 mg/ day in 2-4 divided doses.
*   Doxycycline: 1st day 100 mg at 12 hourly intervals, followed by 100 mg daily.
*   Minocycline: Adults 200 mg to start with, then 100-200 mg once daily.

Adverse drug reactions

*   Tetracyclines possess chelating property. They form calcium tetracycline chelates, which are deposited in growing teeth and bone. If it is given from midpregnancy to 5th month of extrauterine life, ill formed teeth (brown decolouration) are seen, which are more susceptible to form carries. If it is given during 3 months to 5 years of age, the permanent anterior dentition is affected. Similarly, if tetracyclines are used during late pregnancy or childhood, they can cause inhibition of bone growth, which is of course temporary but

there is a chance of bone deformity and height reduction if used for a long period of time.

• Tetracycline, by inducing negative nitrogen balance, can increase blood urea. It depresses protein synthesis and exerts a general catabolic action.

• Demeclocycline may reduce the concentrating capacity of kidney by antagonizing ADH.

• Minocycline may cause vestibular toxicity which disappears on discontinuation of drug.

• Other occasional side effects include hepatic damage, phototoxicity, kidney toxicity (particularly in patients with existing renal disease), hypersensitive reaction, superinfection, etc.

Precautions

• As has already been discussed, tetracyclines are better avoided in children.

• If by mistake expired medicine is used it may produce reversible 'Fancony syndrome'. This is due to damage to proximal tubules caused by degradation products like anhydrotetracycline, epitetracycline and epianhydrotetracycline.

• If tetracycline and penicillin are mixed in a single syringe, inactivation of drugs occurs.

• If used with diuretics, rise in blood urea may occur.

• They should be very cautiously used in renal and hepatic insufficiency cases.

• Tetracycline should not be injected intrathecally.

• Tetracycline is totally contraindicated in pregnant and lactating mothers.

Drug interactions

• Milk and milk products reduce its efficacy.

• Antacids, iron-containing preparations may hamper its absorption.

• Cimetidine decreases its absorption.

- Activity of oral contraceptives is reduced due to decreased potency as tetracyclines disturb the drug carriage system through enterohepatic circulation.
- Tetracyclines increase the hypoprothrombinaemic action of anticoagulants.
- If used concurrently with methoxyflurane, nephrotoxicity of both compounds may supervene.
- Tetracyclines increase the serum level of digoxin.

Macrolides

All macrolide antibiotics possess a large lactone ring in their chemical structure. Important members of this group are erythromycin, roxithromycin, clarithromycin, azithromycin, spiramycin, etc.

Mechanism of action

All macrolides inhibit protein synthesis in bacteria by binding to 50S ribosomal subunit.

Spectrum of activity

Erythromycin acts powerfully on Streptococcus pyogenes, gonococcus, pneumococcus, diphtheria bacillus, clostridia group and listeria. At present, most of the staphylococci and streptococci are resistant towards erythromycin. Other erythromycin-sensitive organisms include mycoplasma, campylobacter, legionella, gardenerella vaginalis, etc. Organisms moderately sensitive to erythromycin are meningococcus, rickettsia, chlamydia trachomatis, B.pertussis, H.influenzae, H. ducreyi, Streptococcus viridans, etc. Roxithromycin has the same spectrum as erythromycin, but is more potent against Gard. vaginalis, legionella, etc., and less potent against B.pertussis.

Clarithromycin, in addition to possessing the spectrum of activity of erythromycin, also possesses power to fight against Mycopacterium avium complex, Mycobacterium leprae, Moraxella, Mycoplasma, H. pylori, etc. Azithromycin has extra powerful action against H. influenzae, Moraxella, chlamydia, gonococcus, etc. Spiramycin inhibits transplacental transmission of toxoplasma gondii infection.

Mechanism of resistance development

Resistance to the drug is developed by:
(a) Production of an enzyme called erythromycin esterase.
(b) Decreased permeability of bacterial membrane to the drug.
(c) Altering of the ribosomal binding site for erythromycin by plasmid encoded methylase enzyme.
(d) Chromosomal mutation causing change in 50S ribosomal subunit.

Cross resistance

Cross resistance between erythromycin and other macrolids, chloramphenicol, clindamycin, etc., has been observed. Possibly, the reason is the close situation of the ribosomal binding sites of these compounds.

Therapeutic uses in ophthalmology

Ocular penetration of erythromycin is poor. This drug can substitute tetracycline in chlamydial and mycoplasma infection in children. Spiramycin is effective against toxoplasmosis. It has been tried in toxoplasmosis during pregnancy. Similarly, azithromycin has been found to produce beneficial action against toxoplasmosis, trachoma, and borreliosis. Roxithromycin has been proven to be effective against mycoplasma and chlamydial infection.

Clarithromycin is a relatively new agent which has been found to be effective against borrelia, nontubercular mycobacteria and Chlamydia, etc.

Preparation and dosage

- Erythromycin tab.: Adults 250-500 mg 3 to 4 times a day; children 30-50 mg/kg/day in divided doses. A topical ointment 3% and lotion 2% are also available for local skin conditions like boil, furuncle, carbuncle, acne vulgaris; etc.
- Roxithromycin: Adults 150 mg twice/day, 15 minutes before meals; children 2.5 to 5 mg/kg/day in two divided doses (not to be used for more than 10 days).
- Azithromycin: Adults 500 mg once daily × 3 days; children 5-10 mg/kg/day × 3 days.

- Spiramycin: Adults 3 million I.U. (MIU) twice daily (for general infections); 6-9 MIU in 2-4 divided doses for toxoplasmosis associated with pregnancy.
- Clarithromycin: Adults 250-500 mg twice daily × 7 days to 14 days; children 15 mg/kg/day in 2 divided doses × 7-14 days.

Contraindications

Hypersensitivity, cross-hypersensitivity may exist between the members of this group.

Precautions

- Hepatic dysfunction.
- Prolonged use should be avoided.
- In case of azithromycin, renal dysfunction and existence of pseudo membranous colitis should also be taken into consideration.

Adverse effects

- G.I. tract irritation may occur.
- Reversible type of hearing impairment may occur if used in very high doses.
- Hypersensitive reactions include drug rash, drug fever, and in case of estolate ester of erythromycin reversible cholestatic jaundice may occur.
- Clarithromycin sometimes produces anaphylaxis, involvement of C.N.S. (insomnia, confusion, etc.) and Stevens Johnson syndrome.

Drug interactions

- It inhibits the oxidation of various drugs in liver resulting in their elevated levels. These drugs include carbamazepine, warfarin, theophylline, valproate, cisapride, terfenadine, astemizole, etc. Of these, high levels of cisapride, terfenadine and astemizole have precipitated death due to ventricular arrythmias.
- Concurrent administration of ergot alkaloids may lead to features of acute toxicity like peripheral ischaemia.

- Serum levels of digoxin may be elevated on concurrent administration of macrolides.
- Clarithromycin decreases steady state Zidovudine level in patients with HIV infection.

Aminoglycosides

These are a group of antibiotics obtained from soil actinomycetes. The first among this group to be discovered was streptomycin, obtained from Streptomyces griseus, and netilmicin, a derivative of sisomicin, is the latest in this group. Streptomycin (Fig.5.10), the first clinically useful antitubercular drug, was discovered by Prof. Selman A. Waksman in 1944 for which he was awarded Nobel Prize in 1952. Chemically, all the members of this group consist of two or more amino sugars linked glycosidically to a hexose nucleus. Important members of this group are: (a) streptomycin, (b) gentamycin, (c) kanamycin, (d) tobramycin, (e) amikacin, (f) sisomicin, (g) netilmicin and (h) neomycin.

Characteristics

- These compounds are not absorbed orally as they ionize in solution and their CSF penetrating capacity is poor. But they can cross the placental barrier.

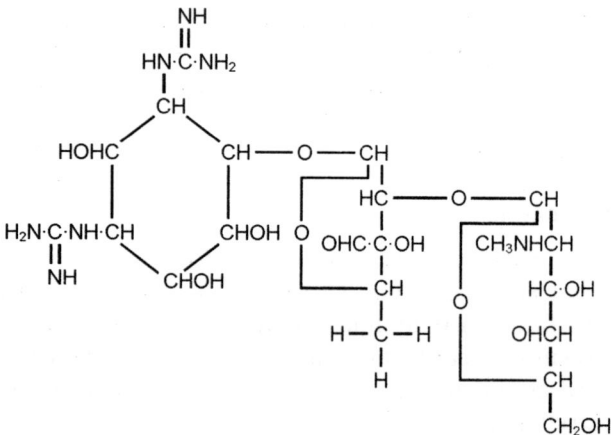

Fig. 5.10. Chemical structure of streptomycin

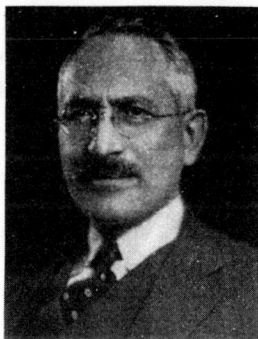

Fig. 5.11. Selman A. Waksman – discoverer of streptomycin

- All these compounds are bactericidal in nature and act best at alkaline pH.
- All of them possess diverse spectrum of activity but one common characteristic is that the bacteria susceptible to them are aerobic Gram-negative bacteria. Both streptomycin and kanamycin are effective against tubercle bacilli.
- Cross resistance between the members may occur, but it is always partial in nature.
- The route of excretion is kidney in unchanged form.
- All of them possess ototoxic and nephrotoxic property, but the magnitude differs.
- All of them act by inhibiting bacterial protein synthesis.
- Margin of safety is less, which is common to all.

Mechanism of action

It involves two processes:

(a) Carriage of aminoglycosides across the bacterial cell membrane:
This process requires two conditions: (1) oxygen supply and (2) alkaline pH.

(b) Formation of wrong peptide chains due to distortion of mRNA codons:
Aminoglycoside streptomycin gets bound to 30S ribosome whereas others may get bound to 50S ribosome and 30S-50S interface.

The above phenomenon leads to misreading of codes and formation of abnormal peptide chain. So, the cell wall now synthesized is abnormal, which leads to leakage of vital metabolites due to increased permeability. It ultimately leads to death of cell.

Development of resistance

Resistance may occur in the following ways:

1. Aminoglycosides carriage inside the bacterial cell is inhibited.
2. Mutation causes diminished affinity of ribosomal units to combine with the concerned drug.
3. There may be inactivation of the drug by some enzymes liberated by microorganisms.

Common side effects

- Ototoxicity: Aminoglycosides may cause progressive destruction of 8th cranial nerve (irreversible in nature). Auditory division is affected by kanamycin, amikacin and neomycin. Vestibular division is affected by streptomycin and gentamycin. Both the divisions may be affected by tobramycin.
- Renal toxicity (reversible in nature): Streptomycin produces minimum and neomycin produces maximum toxicity.
- Neuromuscular blockade: Uncommon in daily practice, but may occur if the aminoglycosides are poured in peritoneal, or pleural membrane (particularly, if curare has been used during anaesthesia in a surgical case). Rapid absorption in these cases may cause neuromuscular blockade leading to apnea and death. However, this action may be partially counteracted by I.V. calcium injection. Neomycin and streptomycin produce this action more commonly than gentamycin, kanamycin and amikacin. Tobramycin is relatively free from this defect. Aminoglycosides should be used with caution in a patient of myasthenia gravis.
- Hypersensitive reactions may sometimes occur. Streptomycin may produce optic nerve damage and paraesthesia.

Role in ophthalmic practice

Neomycin topically produces good effect in Acanthamoeba keratitis. Kanamycin has been proved to be of much value in atypical mycobacteria induced keratitis. Spectinomycin is a little structurally different type of aminoglycoside. Its mechanism of action is also a little different from that of conventional aminoglycosides. It is used mainly in those gonorrhea cases which are either allergic to penicillin or are infected by penicillinase producing gonococci.

Gentamycin is possibly one of the most popular drugs amongst ophthalmologists. A 0.3% solution is commonly used. However, in severe corneal infections, a 2% solution can also be used. If such high concentration is used, efficient concentration is reached in anterior chamber. 20 to 40 mg of gentamycin injection is given subconjunctively (subtenon also), effective bacteriocidal concentration is achieved in deeper tissues of eye. As Pseudomonas group is gradually becoming resistant to gentamycin, nowadays amikacin or ceftazidime are used in cases of intraocular infection. Some ophthalmologists use gentamycin + vancomycin in irrigating fluids during cataract/ vitrectomy/ retinal surgery as a prophylactic measure against bacterial endophthalmitis. This method really provides good prophylaxis against endophthalmitis but is a controversial method. Tobramycin is the drug of choice in Pseudomonas infection. A 0.3% solution is available for topical use. 10-20 mg of subconjunctival injection of tobramycin produces good therapeutic level in anterior chamber (which is retained also for a few hours). Intravitreal injection 100 to 200 microgram has been tried successfully. Sisomicin has a structural and spectral sensitivity resemblance with gentamycin; hence, it is used in gentamycin resistant cases. A 3 mg/ml topical solution is used. Netilmicin is a derivative of sisomicin but its anti-pseudomonas activity is superior to both gentamycin and tobramycin. Amikacin is also a popular drug in ophthalmic practice. It has a structural resemblance with kanamycin. It is used both as a subconjunctival and as an intravitreal injection. It is less toxic to retina than gentamycin; 400 microgram of the drug can be safely used as intravitreal injection. The metabolism rate is higher in inflamed, vitrectomised and aphakic eyes. So, a 2nd dose is often required after 24 to 48 hours. Amikacin is very useful in atypical mycobacterial cases. Framycetin is yet another antibiotic used topically 0.5% eye drop and 1% skin cream. This aminoglycoside is obtained from Streptomycin lavendulae.

Conditions aggravating ototoxicity of aminoglycosides

- Relatively prolonged and repeated therapy.
- Elderly people.
- Concurrent use of diuretics like furosemide and ethacrynic acid.

Conditions potentiating nephrotoxicity of aminoglycosides

(a) Patients with poor renal function.

(b) Patients suffering from dehydration and shock.

(c) Advanced age.

(d) Concurrent administration of drugs like frusemide, cisplatin, vancomycin, cyclosporin, amphotericin B, etc.

Miscellaneous Agents

Clindamycin

It is a derivative of lincomycin (which is usually not used due to its toxicity) belonging to the group of lincosamide antibiotics. Spectrum of activity and mechanism of action are more or less similar to those of erythromycin. Therapeutically, it is mainly used against anaerobes like B. fragilis and in case of mixed infections. It is also used in AIDS patients for the management of toxoplasmosis (along with pyrimethamine) and pneumocystis carinii pneumonia (along with primaquine). The oral dose is 150-300 mg 4 times a day; I.V. dose is 200-600 mg 8 hourly. Topical skin ointment (1%) is also available.

Milder side effects include skin rashes, drug fever, urticaria, pain abdomen. Serious side effects are diarrhoea and pseudomembranous enterocolitis caused by resistant type of Clostridium difficile superinfection. This type of superinfection usually leads to death unless urgently treated with vancomycin (alternatively metronidazole). In ocular toxoplasmosis, clindamycin has been used as subtenon injection (150 mg). It is also used as intravitreal injection (1 mg).

It is contraindicated if hypersensitive reaction occurs. Special precaution is taken in cases of prolonged use (by monitoring LFT, RFT, blood counts).

Drug interactions

- Antagonizes erythromycin.
- Enhances the action of d-tubocurarine.
- Antagonizes neostigmine and pyridostigmine

Vancomycin

It is a very important antibiotic. Its use should be restricted as indiscriminate use may lead to bacterial resistance. In modern ophthalmic practice, it is the drug of choice for intravitreal injection in bacterial endophthalmitis (dose is 1.00 mg) along with an aminoglycoside antibiotic or ceftazidime. It can also be used in vitrectomy cases (in the irrigation fluid) in the concentration of 30 microgram per ml. and in cases of cataract surgery in the concentration 50 to 100 microgram per ml. Anterior and posterior chamber injection of 1 mg of vancomycin produces beneficial results without any problem. It is an antibiotic obtained from a soil actinomycetes Streptomyces orientalis. Chemically, it is a glycopeptide. It acts by inhibition of synthesis of cell wall of sensitive organisms. It gets bound to D-alanyl-D-alanine fraction of the cell wall precursor and produces the damage. It is a bactericidal agent. It is mainly active against Gram-positive bacteria. The spectrum of activity includes various resistant types of Staphylococcus aureus organisms (including methicillin resistant variety), Enterococci, Streptococcus viridans, Clostridium difficile, Neisseria group, diphtheroids, etc. It is not absorbed orally but is used by oral route (250-500 mg 6 hourly) for management of pseudomembranous enterocolitis (a life threatening situation). For systemic diseases, it is used parenterally – 500 mg every 6 hours or 1 g every 12 hours I.V. (the drug should be injected at very slow rate extending over a period of 1 hour). However, the dose should be reduced in renal deficiency diseases. It is a very useful drug for controlling infection in patients undergoing cancer chemotherapy and dialysis and as penicillin substitute in penicillin allergic patients. It is a potentially toxic drug and nephrotoxicity/ ototoxicity is usually dose-dependent. When drugs like aminoglycosides are required for concurrent administration (as a life saving treatment), the dose of individual compounds should be correctly assessed. Other toxic reactions include dermal allergy, thrombophlebitis, intense flush (red man syndrome), sudden fall of blood pressure, etc.

Drug interactions

- Enhancement of action of d-tubocurarine.
- Anion exchange resins like cholestyramine antagonize oral vancomycin.
- Concurrent administration of aminoglycosides increases the risk of nephrotoxicity.

Teicoplanin

It is a newer addition to the list of glycopeptide antibiotics. It is more powerful and possibly less toxic than vancomycin. One additional advantage over vancomycin is that it can be administrated I.M. (400-600 mg I.M. to start with and then 200 mg/day).

Sodium Fusidate

It is a steroidal antibiotic. It exhibits both bacteriostatic and bactericidal properties. It is effective mainly against many Gram-positive bacteria by inhibiting protein synthesis in bacteria. A 2% skin cream is available for local use in skin condition like carbuncles, furuncles, boils, etc. Precaution should be taken so that it is not applied in the eyes. Recently, an eye drop (1%) has been introduced for treatment of bacterial conjunctivitis (used twice daily).

Mupirocin

It is an antibiotic obtained from Pseudomonas fluorescens. It is active against both Gram-positive and -negative organisms infecting skin. A 2% skin ointment is used to treat superficial dermatological conditions caused by staphylococci and streptococci. It is also effective against methicillin resistant Staph. aureus. Contact with eye and nasal mucous membrane is to be avoided.

Spectinomycin

It is an antibiotic derived from Streptomyces spectabillis. Chemically, it resembles aminoglycosides. It is effective against many Gram-negative bacteria. But development of drug resistance is a problem. At present, it is only indicated in penicillinase producing gonococcal infection and penicillin sensitive persons (suffering from gonorrhoea), particularly if the patient is pregnant (where fluoroquinolones are contraindicated). In cases of uncomplicated urethritis, a single dose of 2 g I.M. is sufficient. But in complicated cases, a three-day course is required.

Polypeptide Antibiotics

These include polymyxin B, polymyxin E (Colistin), bacitracin, and tyrothricin.

Polymyxin

Polymyxin B is isolated from Bacillus polymyxa and polymyxin E (Colistin) is isolated from Bacillus colistinus. They are mainly active against Gram-negative bacteria except Proteus, Neisseria group and Serratia. Colistin has been found to be more active than polymyxin B against Pseudomonas, Shigella and Salmonella.

These drugs act as cationic detergents. Due to their high affinity for phospholipids, these agents penetrate and destroy the cellular biology of the microorganism. Thus, they are bacteriocidal agents. They are usually used with other agents to get synergistic action. As these drugs are neurotoxic and nephrotoxic (if administered parenterally), they are usually used as topical agents. In ophthalmology, following combinations of polymyxin B are very popular:

- Polymyxin B + neomycin + gramicidin drop and ointment
- Polymyxin B + Bacitracin drop and ointment
- Polymyxin B + neomycin ointment
- Polymyxin B + trimethroprim eye drop.

Bacitracin

It is a peptide antibiotic isolated from Bacilus subtilis. It is mainly active against Gram-positive cocci and bacilli. It acts by inhibiting the synthesis of bacterial cell wall. Hence, it is a bactericidal agent. It is used only as a topical agent. In ophthalmic practice it has been observed to produce brilliant response in staphylococcal blepharo conjunctivitis. Usually, ointments containing 500 units are available commercially.

Tyrothricin

It is a mixture of two antibiotics – gramicidin and tyrocidine obtained from Bacillus bravis. It is active against many Gram-positive and a few Gram-negative bacteria. It causes leakage of cell membrane of bacteria and thus causes lysis of cells. It is mainly used as a skin cream (0.5 mg/g) for dermal bacterial infections.

Metronidazole

It belongs to the group of nitroimidazole. It is active against protozoal diseases like amoebiasis, trichomoniasis, giardiasis, etc. It is active against many anaeorobic bacteria like Clostridium perfringens, Helicobacter pylori, B fragilis, anaerobic streptococci, Fusobacterium, etc. It facilitates the expulsion of Dracanculus medinensis from skin. It has practically no action against aerobic bacteria.

Mechanism of action

It is not yet well understood. In susceptible microorganisms it enters inside the cell by the process of diffusion. Then its nitro group (Fig. 5.12) is reduced with the formation of intermediate compounds. These compounds probably damage cellular DNA and causes cell death. As it is highly active against anaerobes, it has been suggested that it interferes with electron transport from NADPH or other types of reduced substrates. Metronidazole has been found experimentally to produce mutagenesis (particularly in rodents). It has also been found to depress the cell mediated immunity and to cause radio-sensitization.

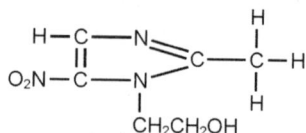

Fig. 5.12. Chemical structure of metronidazole

Side effects

Metronidazole may cause very mild headache, nausea, metallic taste, etc. If used for a prolonged period, neurological manifestations are seen.

Drug interactions

Important drug interactions are:
  (a) Metronidazole produces disulfiram-like action if taken with alcohol.
  (b) Drugs like cimetidine decrease the metabolism of metronidazole.
  (c) Its pharmacological actions may be reduced if taken with enzyme inducers like phenobarbitone, rifampin, etc
  (d) Renal excretion of lithium is decreased if metronidazole is concurrently administered.
  (e) Potentiation of oral anticoagulants like warfarin as a result of which prothrombin time is increased.

Dosage

Usual adult dose is 200-400 mg thrice daily; I.V. infusion 100 ml 8 hourly. 1% gel is used twice daily in facial rosacea.

Antiseptics

Silver nitrate 1% solution is a powerful antibacterial agent, particularly against gonococcus. It has no antiviral property. Povidone – iodine 5% solution is an effective antiseptic compound. Zinc sulphate eye drop 0.1% is effective against diplobacillary conjunctivitis (angular conjunctivitis). In Acanthamoeba infection of eye, chlorhexidine (0.02%) and polyhexamethylene biguanide (0.01% to 0.02%) give good results.

Some Recently Developed Drugs

Some of the recently developed drugs are linezolid, dalfopristin plus quinupristin combination, etc., which require special mention as they are used in Methicillin as well as Vancomycin resistant Staphylococcus aureus (VRSA). Linezolid is an oxazolidinone derivative which is bacteriostatic in nature. It is found to be effective against VRSA. The details of these drugs are beyond the scope of this book.

CHAPTER 6

Antivirals

As viruses are obligatory intracellular parasites, it is very difficult to synthesize a drug which can destroy only virus without injuring the host cell. Moreover, a drug in laboratory animals may be highly specific to a particular virus but in human beings it may not be as effective. However, some of the clinically important antivirals available are as follows:

(1) *Drug used against herpes virus*: Idoxuridine (IDU), Triflurothymidine (Trifluridine), Vidarabine, Ethyldeoxyuridine (Edoxuridine), Acyclovir (ACV), Famcyclovir, Ganciclovir, Foscarnet, etc.

(2) *Drugs used against retrovirus*:
   (a) Nucleoside reverse transcriptase inhibitors (NRTIs), e.g., Zidovudine (AZT), Stavudine (d4T), Didanosine, Zalcitabine, Lamivudine, etc.
   (b) Non-nucleoside reverse transcriptase inhibitors (NNRTIs), e.g., Efavirenz, Nevirapine, etc.
   (c) Drugs acting by protease inhibition, e.g., Indinavir, Ritonavir, Saquinavir, Nelfinavir, etc.

(3) *Drugs acting against influenza virus:* Amantadine, Rimantadine, Tromantadine.

(4) *Miscellaneous anti-viral agents:* Interferon, Ribavirin, Methisazone, Cidofovir, Carbocyclic oxetanocin, Immunoglobulins, etc.

Drugs Used against Herpes Virus

Idoxuridine (IDU)

It was the first virustatic agent which was successfully used in clinical practice. It is 5-iodo-2-deoxyuridine and its chemical structure

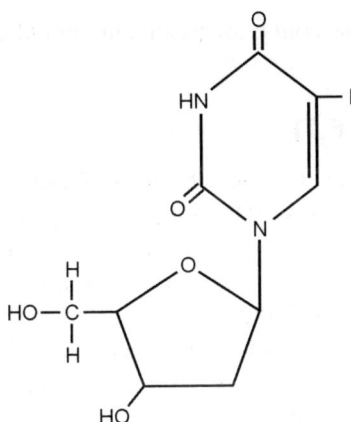

Fig. 6.1. Chemical structure of idoxuridine

(Fig. 6.1) is similar to thymidine. Initially, it is phosphorylated by viral thymidine kinase. It is taken up by the viral DNA by mistake (in place of thymidine) and this phenomenon leads to production of abnormal mRNA. As a result, faulty protein synthesis occurs. Its therapeutic value is confined to Herpes simplex keratitis as a topical agent (systemic administration may lead to bone marrow depression). The drug is not effective in deep stromal keratitis.

Side effects

- Hypersensitive reaction to the chemical substance. There may be allergic blepharitis, thickening of conjunctiva, etc.
- Toxic reactions of the drug molecule include superficial punctate erosions of cornea, follicle formation in conjunctiva, punctum block, conjunctival scarring, etc.
- IDU, being incorporated in both viral and host DNA, is a toxic substance.

Preparation and dosage

It is available as 0.1% eye drop and 0.5% eye ointment. The common line of treatment in dendritic ulcer is as follows:

0.1% solution every 1 to 2 hours during waking period and 0.5% eye ointment at bedtime. Alternatively, 0.5% eye ointment can be used 5 times a day. The course of treatment should not exceed 3 weeks.

Trifluorothymidine (F₃T)

Triflurorothymidine (Fig. 6.2) is a highly effective drug against epithelial herpetic keratitis. Like IDU, it is also initially phosphorylated by viral thymidine kinase (also to some extent by host thymidine kinase). It inhibits cellular thymidylate synthetase resulting in blockage of synthesis of DNA. Moreover, it gets incorporated in the viral DNA and the viral particles lose their infective property. It has been observed that if the drug is used properly, the cure rate in epithelial herpetic keratitis is 90% to 95% within one week.

Preparation and dosage

It is available as 1% drop and 2% ointment. In dendrite ulcer, 1% drop is used 5 to 9 times a day and 2% ointment at night. The course of treatment should not exceed 3 weeks.

Side effects are similar to those in the case of IDU.

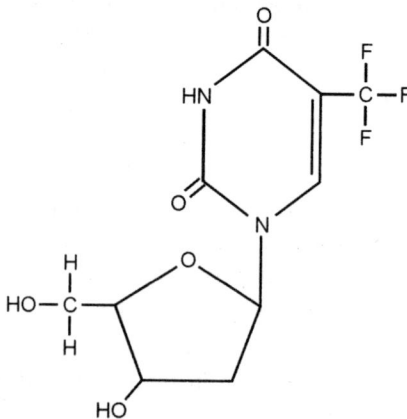

Fig. 6.2. Chemical structure of trifluorothymidine

Vidarabine

Vidarabine (Fig. 6.3) is a purine derivative. It does need the help of viral thymidine kinase to get phosphorylated. Hence, it is a drug of

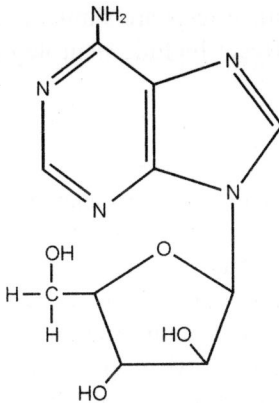

Fig. 6.3. Chemical structure of vidarabine

choice in the management of thymidine kinase deficient mutants of herpes simple virus, where acyclovir is also ineffective. Further, it inhibits both DNA polymerase and RNA reductase. The triphosphate derivative is also sometimes engulfed in the viral DNA and there it acts as a chain terminator. Effective virustatic concentration is achieved in corneal epithelium, stroma and aqueous humour.

Therapeutic uses

- Herpes simplex keratitis: 3% ointment 5 times a day x 3 weeks. Usually, 80-90% cases are cured within 2 weeks.

- Herpes virus induced uveitis resistant to drugs, Herpes simplex encephalitis and Herpes Zoster: The drug is used systemically in the aforesaid conditions. The usual dosage is 10 to 20 mg/kg of body weight to be injected in drip which runs for about 8 to 10 hours. In life threatening cases, treatment for 10 days is usually required.

Cytarabine

It is an antiviral agent effective against Herpes simplex and Ocular Vaccinia. It acts by inhibiting nucleic acid synthesis. The usual preparations available are eye drop (0.5-1%) and eye ointment (1%). It can also be used systemically in the dose 30-100 mg/m^2/day intravenously. Ocular side effects are similar to those in the case of IDU. Systemic side effects include neurological manifestations, myalgia, leucopenia, etc.

Ethyl Deoxyuridine

It is also known as edoxuridine. It is selectively activated by viral thymidine kinase. It acts by inhibiting DNA polymerase. It is more effective against HSV 2 than 1; hence, it is more useful in genital herpes. However, HSV keratitis responds well to it. Even subconjunctival and systemic administration is possible. Side effects are practically nil. Usually, 2% eye drop (5 to 8 times) a day and 0.3% eye gel (to be used at bed time) are available.

Acyclovir

It is structurally similar to purine nucleoside (Fig. 6.4).

Mechanism of action

The initial step is its activation by viral thymidine kinase to acyclovir monophosphate, which thus occurs specifically in virus infected cells; other host cells are practically not affected by this reaction. Next, the drug penetrates deeply in the viral infected cells. The final activation product, acyclovir triphosphate, has approximately 30 times greater affinity for viral DNA polymerase, which it depresses, than host normal cell DNA polymerase. The moment the final activated product enters the viral DNA chain everything collapses and the virus is killed.

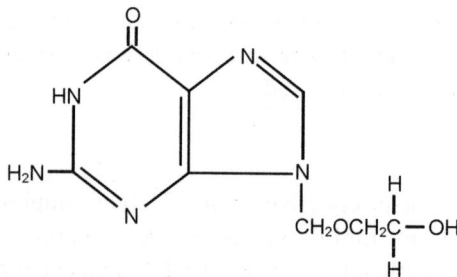

Fig. 6.4. Chemical structure of acyclovir

It is active both topically and systemically. Since the absorption is slow, effective concentration is not reached quickly. After a few days, the virus shows resistance to the drug. The mechanism of resistance may be as follows:

- Virus stops to produce thymidine kinase.
- Altered type of thymidine kinase forms, which bypasses the drug.
- Structural derangement of viral DNA polymerase.

Clinical use

- It has been successfully used topically in management of herpes simplex keratitis and herpes zoster uveitis. Deep stromal lesions also respond well to it. As it is less host cell toxic, it can be used for a prolonged period.
- It has been successfully used topically, orally and intravenously in the management of Herpes Zoster Ophthalmicus.
- It has also been found effective in the management of mucocutaneous herpes, genital herpes and cerebral herpes. Chicken pox in immuno-compromised patients also responds well.
- Prophylactic use of oral acyclovir has reduced many incidences of relapse of herpetic keratitis in corneal graft cases.

Adverse reactions

- Topically, it is a remarkable non-toxic drug. In a few cases conjunctival irritation and superficial punctate erosions may occur.
- Systemically, in low therapeutic doses a little headache, nausea, diarrhoea, dermal allergy, etc., may occur. Very rarely, renal damage may occur. With relatively higher doses, particularly when used I.V., slight neurological manifestations like tremor, disorientation of space and time, etc., may occur.

Available preparations with doses

- 3% ophthalmic ointment – 5 times a day, to be continued for a minimum period of 3 days after clinical healing.

- A 5% ointment is available for treatment of genital herpes. It is also useful in recurring herpes in immuno-compromised patients.
- Oral dose for superficial herpetic keratis is 200 mg 5 times a day. For Herpes Zoster, 800 mg 5 times a day; and for herpetic iritis, 400 mg 5 times a day. For prophylactic use in prevention of herpes recurrence on corneal grafts, 800 mg per day has been suggested. The extent of treatment is limited to 2-8 weeks. In case of renal hypofunction, the dose is decreased and in case of malabsorption, the dose may be increased according to need.
- Intravenous dose for herpetic encephalitis is 30 mg/kg/day in 3 divided doses for 10 days. In acute retinal necrosis the dose suggested is 10-15 mg/kg thrice daily I.V. x 10-14 days.
- Intravitreal dose is 80 to 160 microgram.

Valacyclovir

Valcyclovir is a pro drug of acyclovir. After absorption in the body, it is converted to its active ingredient which has an antiviral potency about 3 to 4 times more than that achieved by oral acyclovir. In preventing relapse of genital herpes, it is used orally as 0.5 g twice daily, which is equivalent to 200 mg acyclovir taken 5 times a day. In case of Herpes Zoster infection, a dose of 1 g is given orally, thrice daily for 10 days.

Famciclovir

Famciclovir is a pro drug of penciclovir. On oral administration, it achieves a bioavailability of 77% compared to acyclovir which achieves a bioavailability of 15 to 20%. It has been successfully used in HSV Keratitis (125 mg B.D. orally) and Herpes Zoster and Varicella infection (500 mg thrice daily orally for 10 days).

Ganciclovir

It is chemically related to acyclovir. The drug is activated to monophosphorylate ganciclovir by the enzyme deoxyguanosine kinase present in cytomegalovirus (CMV). Of course, some phosphorylation takes place in uninfected cells also by the enzymes present in the cell.

Monophosphorylate ganciclovir inhibits the CMV DNA polymerase. Additionally, it acts as a faulty substrate for CMV DNA polymerase. All these reactions lead to destruction of virus. Host cell polymerase is also affected, but to a lesser extent due to lesser affinity of the phosphorylated compound for host cell DNA polymerase. Clinically, it is successfully used in the management of CMV retinitis in immunocompromised patients and Herpes Simplex Keratitis. In CMV retinitis, it is initially given 3.5-5 mg/kg of body weight twice daily I.V. for 10-20 days. Then the maintenance dose given is 5 mg/kg of body weight once daily I.V. infusion extending for a period of 1 hour for 7 days. Lastly, an oral maintenance dose is followed, 1 g thrice daily with food. Ganciclovir can be used as intravitreal injection; the dose is 2 mg. An intraocular sustained release preparation is available which contains 4.5 mg of the drug and the release rate is one microgram per hour for a period 6 months. For the management of Herpes Simplex Keratitis, a topical gel (0.15%) is used 5 times a day.

Adverse reactions

The basic adverse reaction is reversible neutropenia. This can be counteracted by stimulating leucopoesis with the help of granulocyte macrophage colony stimulating factor (GM-CSF). Anemia may also occur which is managed by erythropoetin. Other side effects include thrombocytopenia, mental confusion, drug rash, drug fever, etc. However, if in spite of all measures the neutrophilic leucocyte count goes below 500/ml or platelet count goes below 25,000/ml, the therapy should be immediately stopped.

Foscarnet

It is a drug which inhibits replication of all types of herpes viruses (infecting human beings) and retroviruses (which include HIV). It selectively inhibits viral DNA polymerase and reverse transcription by blocking the pyrophosphate binding site of these enzymes. The drug is active against acyclovir-resistant viruses as it does not require any preliminary activation (phosphorylation). The main therapeutic use of foscarnet (Fig. 6.5) is in (a) CMV infection of severe type, (b) mucocutaneous herpes of AIDS, resistant to acyclovir. Initially, a dose of 60 mg per kg body weight 8 hourly x 2-3 weeks is started.

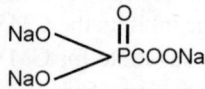

Fig. 6.5. Chemical structure of foscarnet

This is followed by 120 mg/kg body weight once daily to be continued till required. It is usually used in combination with Zidovudin in AIDS as there is no neuropenia problem with it. Dose adjustment is done in patients with renal insufficiency. Correction of fluid balance by I.V. infusion is of paramount importance. In severe cases, it can be used intravitreally, 2.4 mg in 0.1 ml solution only once a week.

Its side effects include phlebitis, nephrotoxicity, neurological manifestations (tremors), elevation of hepatic enzyme levels, fall in calcium, magnesium and phosphate level, anemia, etc.

Drugs Used against Retrovirus

Zidovudine

Chemically, it is azidothymidine (AZT) (Fig. 6.6). In human immunodeficiency virus, it inhibits viral reverse transcriptase. So, the production of viral DNA chains is prevented. Host cell DNA polymerase does not possess that much affinity for it as the viral reverse transcriptase. Once it enters inside the DNA molecules, it functions as DNA chain terminator.

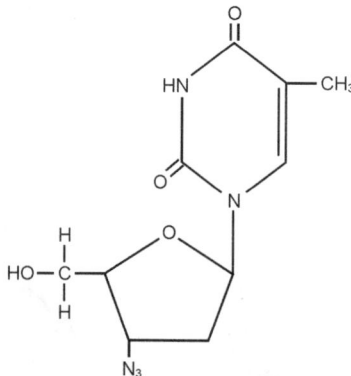

Fig. 6.6. Chemical structure of Zidovudine

Its bioavailability is about 65% after oral administration. It is mainly excreted as glucoronide but some percentage (15-20%) is excreted unchanged. It can cross the placental barrier and it is found in milk also. When used in AIDS, it prolongs life, induces a sense of well being and also resists opportunistic infections. But it cannot cure the disease. After a time (from a few months to two years), the virus becomes refractory to this drug. The most important side effects are neutropenia and anemia and so frequent blood transfusion, G-CSF, GM-CSF, erythropoetin therapy are needed. Other features are G.I. tract irritation, myalgia, headache, etc., but these features usually diminish after continuation of treatment.

Concurrent administration of paracetamol, azole antifungal may increase the toxicity of AZT. Some other drugs like myelo suppressives, probenecid, etc., may also increase its toxicity.

The usual recommended dose in adults is 500 mg per day in two to four divided doses.

Other Nucleoside Reverse Transcriptase Inhibitors (NRTIS)

These include lamivudine, stavudine, didanosine, zalcitabine, etc., which are all viral reverse transcriptase inhibitors. They may show activity against zidovudine-resistant cases. But when used alone all of them become refractory after some time.

Non-nucleoside Reverse Transcriptase Inhibitors (NNRTIS)

These are newer additions in the management of AIDS. Two drugs are used clinically – efavirenz and nevirapine. These do not need to go for intracellular phosphorylation for their antiviral action. These can directly suppress HIV reverse transcriptase.

Protease Inhibitors

These compounds (PI) are again the result of research against AIDS. It has been observed that the enzyme aspartic protease plays an important role in the life cycle of HIV in the production of its structural protein and other metabolites. Four compounds possessing anti-protease activity have been found to be clinically beneficial in the management of AIDS. They are indinavir, ritonavir, saquinavir and nelfinavir. These drugs prevent the maturation of newly developed virus particles by blocking the late step of HIV replication (for which aspartic protease is needed). As a result, a new generation of non-infectious virus particles are produced which possess much reduced reverse transcriptase activity. So, if this group of drugs is added with zidovudine group, they act synergistically. The important side effects of this group include G.I. host irritation, exacerbation of diabetes, asthenia, headache, etc.

Guidelines for management of AIDS

The treatment should be started before CD4 count falls below 200 per microlitre. Another important parameter is HIV-RNA level. When it is more than 50 thousand copies per ml, it is accepted as high level and the treatment should be started. When the treatment is started it should be HAART, i.e., highly active anti-retroviral therapy which usually includes combination therapy comprising three drugs. It may include two nucleoside reverse transcriptase inhibitors (NRTIs) along with a protease inhibitor, or two NRTIs along with a non-nucleoside reverse transcriptase inhibitor (NNRTI) or a combination of three NRTIs.

Drugs Used in Influenza A Virus

Amantadine is the classical drug used against influenza A virus. It is also used as an anti-parkinsonian agent. As far as antiviral activity is concerned, it inhibits the un-coating of virus and also prevents its further penetration into host cells. The adsorption of virus is not affected. Under these circumstances, the host cell antibodies attack the virus and inactivate them. It is usually well tolerated. Milder side effects include ataxia, nightmares, insomnia, postural hypotension, ankle edema, etc. It is contraindicated in neurological diseases (like epilepsy), during pregnancy and in presence of peptic ulcer. The usual dose is 100 mg twice daily. Other drugs of this group are rimantadine and tromantadine. The latter is believed to possess activity against herpes simplex infection.

Miscellaneous Anti-viral Agents

Interferon

Chemically, it is a glycoprotein and immunologically, it offers a non-specific type of immune defence against viral infections. Interferons are produced by virus infected host cells. They mainly belong to three groups:

(a) Alpha-interferons: These are derived from lymphocytes and macrophages. Fifteen subtypes have been recognized. These stimulate the production of antibodies and have been found to be helpful in B cell differentiation also.

(b) Beta-interferons: These are derived from epithelial cells and fibroblasts. Two subtypes have been recognized "Beta one" and "Beta two". Beta one interferon activates natural killer cells and it has also been found to inhibit viral replication. Beta two interferon is also called interleukin (IL-6).

(c) Gamma-interferon: This is derived from T lymphocytes and helps the immune mechanism in identifying the viral antigens.

Mechanism of action

Interferons increase the effectiveness of natural killer cells and phagocytic property of macrophages. Their formation is induced by many viruses particularly RNA type. After their formation, they stimulate the surface receptor cells of the host to produce antiviral enzyme, which suppresses viral transcription and translation. Synthesis and release are also found to be inhibited. But properties like uncoating adhesion, deeper penetration, etc., are not affected. Ultimately, there is inhibition of viral replication.

Apart from their antiviral property, interferons have many other functions which include:

(a) Stimulating activity of macrophage induced phagocytosis, natural killer cell and cytotoxic T cells.

(b) Antineoplastic activity, as suggested by their antagonistic activity against lymphocyte induced and tumour induced angiogenesis property.

(c) Interferons have an important role in expression of MHC (major histocompatibility complex) class–I alpha, beta, gamma types and MHC class II only gamma type. Thus, they play a major part in immunomodulation.

Preparations and dosage

- Recombinant interferon alpha 2a is available as injectible solution in vials containing 3 million I.U.
- Gamma interferon is available as lyophilized powder, 1 mg containing 20 million units.

Alpha 2a is initially started with a dose of 3 million I.U. per day. Then the same dose is used thrice per week. Solution is injected either I.M. or subcutaneously. It has also been tried topically, 10 to 30 million units per ml – 1 drop twice daily.

Gamma interferon is used I.M. or subcutaneously, 1 to 10 million units per day per square meter of body surface.

Adverse reactions

When used topically, it may produce local allergy, SPK-like features and intense chemical conjunctivitis. Systemic side effects include muscle pain, hypotension, nausea, influenza-like syndrome, ischaemia, optic neuropathy, hepatic damage, alopecia and reversible type of bone marrow depression.

Therapeutic uses

- *Ophthalmic uses*: It has been used in the management of Herpes simplex keratitis along with other antivirals in immuno-compromised patients. Its role has been extensively studied in various ophthalmic conditions like adenoviral kerato conjunctivitis, Behcet's disease, Grave's disease, CMV retinitis, conjunctival papillomas, etc., but results are not yet fully understood.
- *Non ophthalmic uses*: Interferon alpha is used in Kaposi's Sarcoma (in AIDS), chronic viral hepatitis (type B and C), hairy cell leukaemia and condyloma acuminata (refractory cases). Interferon gamma is used in chronic granulomatous disease conditions as an immunomodulatory agent.

Ribavirin

It is a reverse transcriptase inhibitor. It is used against viral infections of upper respiratory tract (respiratory syncytial cirus) as aerosol in children.

Methisazone

It is orally effective chemical compound which can work against vaccinia and small pox virus, provided it is used within two days after contact with infected patients. The usual dose is 2 to 4 g only.

Cidofovir

It is a broad spectrum antiviral agent. It is effective against Herpes Simplex virus, CMV, Vericella Zoster and oncogenic viruses like papilloma virus and adenoma virus. It does not require viral thymidine kinase for its activation and so is highly effective against mutant strains, where acyclovir type of medicine is ineffective. Its main side effect is renal damage. There is proteinurea and high creatinine level in blood. Ophthalmic side effects are anterior uveitis and ocular hypotonia. Systemic dose is 5 mg/kg of body weight once a week given intravenously for two consecutive weeks. Later on, it is given in alternate weeks. During its therapy, probenecid and I.V. fluid are given. Topically, HSV keratitis and adenoviral kerato conjunctivitis (0.2% solution twice daily in HSV cases and 4 times a day in adenovirus cases) shows promising result. Intravitreal injection, 20 microgram at 6-week intervals, has shown good results in the management of CMV retinitis.

Carbocyclic Oxetanocin

It is a new broad-spectrum antiviral agent. It is effective against HSV, CMV, HIV, HZV, EBV, etc. In ophthalmic practice, a 0.1% solution is used to treat dendritic corneal ulcer, given 5 times a day for 2 weeks.

Immunoglobulins

Immunoglobulins may act in two ways. (i) Since they contain antiviral antibodies, they can act against viral antigen directly. (ii) Whenever a virus enters the human body and infects a cell, immediately it is identified by cytoxic T cells and they destroy the virus-infected cell as a whole. In this way, although the virus is killed, the host cell is also killed along with it. This identification factor may be blocked by the immunoglobulins. Clinically, in ophthalmic practice, immunoglobulins have been tried in CMV retinitis, Kawasaki's disease and vaccinia infections. Topically, these have also been studied in HSV keratitis. Some of the important non-ophthalmic indications of immunoglobulin therapy include viral hepatitis A and B chicken pox, measles, polio, mumps, etc.

CHAPTER 7

Antifungals

In recent years, due to indiscriminate use of strong antibiotics, corticosteroids, immunosuppressive agents, antineoplastic drugs and increasing incidence of AIDS, the incidence of ocular mycotic infections has increased to a great extent.

Common Ocular Myotic Infections

1. Eyelids

(a) Candida albicans infection usually affects lid margins and roots of eye lashes.

(b) Ringworm, caused by Microsporum trichophyton or M. epidermophton may involve the skin of lid.

(c) Rhinosporoidoses caused by Rhinosporidium seeberi (where soft polypoid masses, which bleed when touched, are seen) is also a common infection.

(d) Other fungal infections of lid include pityrosporosis (caused by Pityrosporum ovale and P. orbiculare – associated with seborrheic blepharitis), blastomycosis (caused by Blastomyces dermatitides and B. brasiliensis), cryptococcosis (caused by Cryptococcus neoformans) and coccidioidomycosis (caused by Coccidioides immitis).

2. Conjunctiva

The most common mycotic infection of conjunctiva is caused by Sporotrichum schenckii. Usually the lids and conjunctiva are affected simultaneously. This type of infection is very common amongst agricultural workers and gardeners.

3. Cornea

Kerotomycosis may occur following an ocular trauma and the organisms responsible in these cases are filamentous fungi like Aspergillus, Fusarium, Cephalosporium, etc. Sometimes, a secondary fungal infection caused by Candida is also seen on a pre-existing corneal pathological condition like neuroparalytic keratitis, keratoconjunctivitis sicca and, occasionally, in contact lens users.

4. Orbit

Orbital mycosis is seen in patients with low immune power, e.g., chronic alcoholics, diabetics patients in the terminal stage of malignant disease, patients undergoing immunosuppressive therapy, AIDS patients, etc. The fungi responsible are usually saprophytic, but become virulent under favourbale circumstances, e.g., Rhizopus, Zygomycetes, Phycomycetes, etc.

Classification of Antifungals

1. Antifungal Antibiotics

   (a) Polyene antibiotics: Natamycin, Amphotericin B, Nystatin.
   (b) Heterocyclic benzofuran group: Griseofulvin.

2. Azole Group

   (a) Imidazole compounds: miconazole, clotrimazole, econazole, ketoconazole.
   (b) Triazole compounds: Fluconazole, Itraconazole.

3. Pyrimidine derivatives

Flucytosine.

4. Miscellaneous Agents

Saperconazole, Terconazole, Faerifungin, Terbenafine, Hamycin, Ciclopirox olamine, Tolnaftate, etc.

Important Antifungal Antibiotics

Natamycin

It is a polyene antibiotic useful in Fusarium Solani Keratitis. A 5% eye drop and 1% eye ointment are used clinically. It cannot deeply penetrate the cornea; hence, it is not very much useful in deep fungal infections. In the form of eye drops, 1 drop is administered at one hour intervals throughout the day and night, and then gradually tapered off. The drug has shown very good anti-fungal property against Candida albicans.

Amphotericin – B

It is a polyene antibiotic obtained from Streptomyces nodosus.

Mechanism of action

The polyene group antibiotics attack the sterol group present in cell membranes of sensitive fungi. As a result there is an increased cellular permeability leading to lysis of cell and death. At the same time it also attacks the cholesterol of cell membrane of host (but in lesser magnitude) causing nephrotoxicity.

Antifungal spectrum

Various fungi and yeasts are sensitive to amphotericin B, which include Candida albicans, Blastomyces dermatidis, Histoplasma capsulatum, Cryptococcus neoformans, Aspergillus, Sporothrix, etc. Various species of Leishmania are also sensitive (it is a reserved drug for Kala-azar).

Ocular indications

Mycotic corneal ulcer and mycotic endophthalmitis (both metastatic and exogenous type).

Mode of administration

- *Topical*: Used as eye drop, 0.1% to 1%.

- *Subconjunctival injection*: It is a back dated treatment and it is not in much use now because of local tissue toxicity and poor penetrating capacity into cornea and deeper ocular tissues.
- *Intracameral route*: It is used and has been found to be non-toxic to corneal endothelium in doses of 2.5 to 5 microgram injected into anterior chamber.
- *Intravitreal route*: 5-10 microgram is injected in the vitreous cavity and it has been found to be non-toxic to retina and lens.
- *Parenteral route*: The drug is available as 50 mg vial. It is dissolved in distilled water or 5% glucose. A test dose of 1 mg in 150 ml. of 5% glucose solution is infused. If there is adverse reaction like chill, nausea, rise of temperature, etc., 30 mg of hydrocortisone is added to the infusion. Next, 1-5 mg of the drug is gradually infused extending for 4-6 hours. The dose has to be increased daily, by 5-10 mg every 12 hours, to reach a dose of 0.75 to 1 mg per kg of body weight. The usual course of treatment is 6-12 weeks. Renal function tests should be done at least twice weekly and if there is any problem the treatment is to be discontinued for a few days. Another problem is hypokalemia, which can be treated by potassium supplementation. In fungal meningitis, 0.5 mg twice weekly intrathecal dose gives good results.
- *Oral route*: It is not absorbed orally, but is used for treatment of intestinal moniliasis orally, 50-100 mg QID.

Adverse reactions

- *Immediate*: As has already been mentioned, during each infusion there is attack of chill, rigor, pain all over body, dyspnoea, etc., usually lasting for 2 to 5 hours, which is probably due to release of cytokines (interleukin, tumour necrosis factor also called TNF). However, these can be managed by corticosteroids.
- *Delayed toxicities*: These are nephrotoxicities, bone marrow depression (anaemia), and CNS toxicities (particularly with intrathecal injections).

Drug interactions

- Flucytosine has synergistic action with AMB provided the fungus is sensitive to both.
- Nephrotoxic drugs like aminoglycosides enhance the nephrotoxicity of AMB.
- Antibiotics like rifampin and minocycline potentiate the action of AMB, although they themselves do not possess antifungal property.

Some new preparations

To reduce the overall toxicity, newer preparations have been introduced in the market. These are:
- Amphotericin B colloidal dispersion (ABCD).
- Amphotericin B lipid complex (ABLC).
- Liposomal amphotericin B.
- Amphotericin B methyl ester.

Nystatin

It is the oldest polyene antibiotic obtained from S. noursei. It is mainly used in ophthalmology in the management of Candida conjunctivitis and keratitis. It is available in the market as an eye ointment.

Griseofulvin

Griseofulvin is obtained from Penicillium griseofulvum. It is used systemically in dermatophyte infections. In ophthalmology, it is used in dermetophyte infection involving skin of lids in the neighbourhood of eye. It gets accumulated in keratin forming cells of skin, hair and nails, especially in fungus infected cells. As it is fungistatic (and not fungicidal), it does not allow the infection to spread in newly formed keratin but it is retained in already infected keratin till it is shed off. In the infection of the skin of eyelid, a treatment for 3 weeks is usually sufficient. Side effects are not serious; only headache may be a prominent feature.

Usual dose is 125 to 250 mg QID with meals.

Drug interactions

- It should not be used in alcoholics as it may produce disulfiram like effect.
- Concurrent administration of phenobarbitone may produce failure in therapy as barbiturates reduce its oral absorption and also induce its metabolism.
- Griseofulvin reduces the effectivity of oral contraceptives.
- Griseofulvin causes induction of warfarin metabolism.

Antifungals of Azole Group

Clotrimazole

Clotrimazole (Fig. 7.1) is a very good drug in the management of Acanthamoeba keratitis.

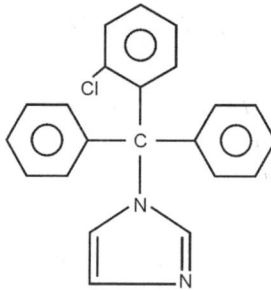

Fig. 7.1. Chemical structure of clotrimazole

Miconazole

It is effective against a wide variety of yeasts and filamentous fungi. Clinically, 1% topical solution and 2% ointment are generally used. Subconjunctival injection, 10 mg, is also used. Intravitreal injection, 20-50 microgram has been used. Systemically, 30 mg/kg of body weight / day given in 3 doses I.V. infusion yields beneficial results.

Ketoconazole

Ketoconazole (Fig. 7.2) is very effective in the management of endogenous uveitis along with cyclosporin. It is regarded as a broad spectrum antifungal agent effective against both dermatophytosis and deep mycosis; it is orally effective. The usual orally effective dose is 200 mg once or twice daily. 2% skin ointment and 2% shampoo are also available.

Side effects

The most important side effect is nausea and vomiting. Other side effects include gynaecomastia, hepatic damage, etc.

Drug interactions

Antacids, H2 blockers and protein pump blockers reduce its oral absorption. Drugs like phenytoin and rifampin induce its metabolism and thereby reduce its efficacy. Ketoconanazole can raise the blood level of cisapride, terfenadine and astemizole and this may lead to fatal ventricular fibrillation. Ketoconazole by depressing the cytochrome P450 raises the blood level of sulfonylureas, phenytoin, cyclosporine, etc.

Contraindication

Ketoconazole is contraindicated in pregnant and nursing women.

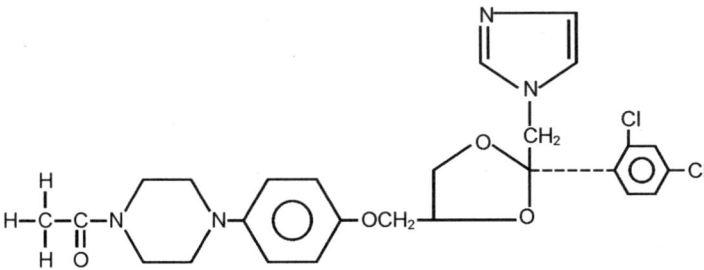

Fig. 7.2. Chemical structure of ketoconazole

Fluconazole

Fluconazole is a triazole compound having a stronger affinity for fungal cytochrome P450 enzymes than human cytochrome P450 enzymes. It is well absorbed through oral route and its absorption is not affected by gastric pH or food. It is very effective against Candida and

Cryptococcus and is a non-toxic drug. Sometimes, nausea, vomiting and abdominal pain may occur.

It is a very good agent in the management of Candida endophthalmitis and other intra-ocular fungal infections. Oral administration produces adequate corneal and anterior chamber concentration. The usual oral dose is 200 to 400 mg per day in divided doses × 4 to 12 weeks. Topically, 0.2% solution is highly effective. Intravitreal Injection 0.1 mg produces a good effect in fungal endophthalmitis. It increases the blood level of sulfonylureas, warfarin, phenytoin, etc.

Pyrimidine Derivatives

Flucytosine

Chemically, it is fluorinated pyrimidine and is converted into 5-fluoruracil in susceptible fungi which interferes with DNA and RNA metabolism of fungus. The conversion of 5FC to 5-fluorauracil is not up to that extent in host cells. Individually it is not a very good drug since resistance develops quickly but as a synergistic agent with AMB, it produces satisfactory result in some cases of ocular candidal infection. 1% topical drug has been used. The average oral dose is 100-150 mg/ kg of body weight/ day in 4 divided doses.

Miscellaneous Agents

Econazole

It is effective against Aspergillosis and Candidiasis. Oral dose is 200 mg tablet thrice daily. It is also available as 1% skin cream.

Itraconazole

It is effective against Candida, Aspergillus and Cryptococcus. Oral dose is 100 to 400 mg per day. 10 microgram intravitreal injection can also be used in endophthalmitis.

Saperconazole

It is a triazole, active against Candida and Aspergillus. A 0.25% solution is used topically and 200 mg tablet once a day is used orally.

Terconazole

It is a new antifungal mainly used as intravitreous injection, 10 to 20 micrograms in 0.1 ml.

Faerifungin

It is a recent antifungal which possesses antibacterial property also. Results of trials in endophthalmitis are encouraging.

Terbenafine

It is an allylamine antifungal and acts by inhibiting the enzyme squalene epoxidase of fungal cell resulting in interference in synthesis of ergosterol, which leads to death of fungal cell. It is a powerful agent against Fusarium.

Hamycin

It is a research product of Hindustan Antibiotics at Pimpri. It is useful in dermal candidiasis.

Ciclopirox olamine

It is effective against dermal candidiasis as 1% solution or cream.

Tolnaftate

Tolnaftate (Fig. 7.3) is a good drug against tinea cruris and taenia corpiris, but is not that much effective against tinea pedis, taenia unguim and tinea capitis. Both, 1% solution and cream are available for dermatological purpose.

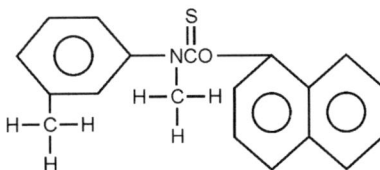

Fig. 7.3. Chemical structure of tolnaftate

CHAPTER 8

Antiparasitic Drugs

A large number of parasitic infestations may involve eye. Important drugs used in ocular parasitic infestations are listed in Table 8.1 below:

Table 8.1. Important groups of parasitic infestations and drugs used

Parasites	Drugs used
A. Protozoa	
I. Amoeba	
(a) Entamoeba histolytica:	Metronidazole, Tinidazole, Secnidazole, Ornidazole, Satranidazole, etc.
(b) Acanthamoeba:	Propamidine isethionate, Neomycin, Clotrimazole, etc.
II. Flagellates	
(a) Giardia lamblia:	Metronidazole, Tinidazole, Furazolidine, Mepacrine, Paromomycin, etc.
(b) Trypanosoma group:	Suramin, Pentamidine, Melarsoprol, Eflornithine, Nifurtimox, etc.
(c) Leishmaniasis	
(i) L. donovani (kala-azar):	Sodium stibogluconate, Antimony meglumine, etc.
(ii) L. tropica (oriental sore):	Pentamidine isethionate
(iii) L. brasiliensis (American mucocutaneous leishmaniasis):	Sodium stibogluconate, Amphotericin B, etc.
III. Sporozoa	
(a) Pneumocystis carinii:	Co-trimoxazole, Pentamidine, etc.

(b) Plasmodium group: Chloroquine, combination of pyrimethamine and ultra-long acting sulfonamides, viz., sulfadoxine, sulfamethopyrazine, quinine, mefloquine, artemisin derivatives like artesunate, artemether, etc.

(c) Toxoplasma gondii: Combination of pyrimethamine and sulfadiazine, clindamycin, atovaquone, etc.

B. Helminths

I. Nematodes

(a) Ascaris lumbricoides: Mebendazole, Piperazine citrate, Pyrantel pamoate, Albendazole, Levamisole, etc.

(b) Enterobius vermicularis: Mebendazole, Pyrantel pamoate, Pyrvinium embonate, Albendazole, etc.

(c) Ankylostoma duodenale and Necator americanus: Pyrantel pamoate, Mebendazole, Albendazole, Bephenium hydroxynephthoate, etc.

(d) Loa loa: Diethylcarbamazine citrate.

(e) Wuchereria group: Ivermactin, Diethylcarbamazine citrate, etc.

(f) Onchocerca group: Ivermactin, Amocarazine, etc.

(g) Dracunculus medinensis: Metronidazole, Thiabendazole, Mebendazole, Niridazole, etc.

(h) Toxocara group: Thiabendazole, Albendazole, Mebendazole, Ivermectin.

(i) Gnathostoma: Albendazole, Mebendazole, etc.

(j) Baylisascaris procyonis: Thiabendazole, Ivermectin

(k) Angiostrongylus cantonensis: Mebendazole, Albendazole, etc.

(l) Trichina spiralis: Thiabendazole, Mebendazole, etc.

(m) Dirofilaria group: Diethylcarbamazine citrate, etc.

(n) Thelazia group: Diethylcarbamazine citrate, etc.

II. Trematodes

(a) Paragonimus westermani: (Lung fluke)	Praziquantel, Bithionol, etc.
(b) Schistosoma group: (Blood flukes)	Praziquantel, Niridazole, etc.
(c) Alaria species:	Albendazole, Praziquantel, etc.

III. Cestodes

(a) Taenia group: (cysticercosis)	Albendazole, Praziquantel, Metrifonate, etc.
(b) Echinococcus species: (hydatidcyst)	Mebendazole, Albendazole, etc.
(c) Coenuris cerebralis:	Praziquantel
(d) Spirometra (sparganosis):	Neoarsphenamine

C. Ectoparasites

I. Tick:	Pilocarpine eye ointment, 4%
II. Louse:	Silver nitrate 1%, yellow mercuric oxide ointment, Physostigmine ointment, Malathion shampoo, etc.
III. Mite:	Ether, Potassium polysulfide, yellow mercuric oxide ointment, etc.
IV. Larvae of flies (Maggots):	Local anaesthetics, Anticholinesterase ointment, Corticosteroids, Antibiotic ointment, NSAIDs, etc.

Some Important Antiparasitic Drugs

Metronidazole

Details have already been discussed in Chapter 5. It is useful against amoebiasis, giardiasis, trichomoniasis and some other conditions like anaerobic bacterial infection, Helicobacter pylori infection, ulcerative gingivitis, pseudo-membranous enterocolitis, etc. Other nitroimidazoles used are tinidazole, ornidazole, secnidazole, satranidazole, etc. Niridazole is the drug of choice in guineaworm infestation.

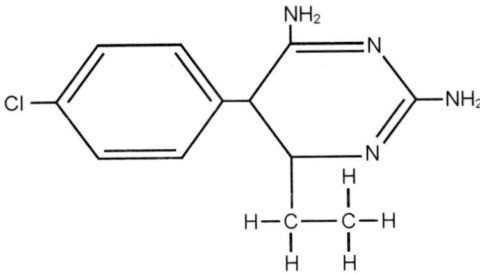

Fig. 8.1. Chemical structure of pyrimethamine

Pyrimethamine

Pyrimethamine (Fig. 8.1) acts by inhibiting the dihydrofolate reductase in Toxoplasma gondii. Folinic acid (which cannot be utilised by the parasite) is given during pyrimethamine therapy (5 mg, thrice a week) to protect the host cells.

Atovaquone

It is a hydroxynaphthoquinone compound which is found to be effective against Pneumocystis carinii, Toxoplasma gondii and Plasmodium group. It interferes with mitochondrial electron transport mechanism of the aforesaid organisms. Fatty foods like butter, cheese, etc., increase the rate of absorption of atovaquone.

Sodium Stibogluconate

It is a pentavalent antimony compound. It is the drug of first choice in kala-azar. Exact mechanism of its action is not understood. Probably it acts by:

- Inhibiting sulfhydryl dependant enzyme system.
- By interfering with fatty acid oxidation and glycolytic pathways.
- Recently, a liposomal delivery system has been developed which is more specific in killing the parasite.

Milder side effects are G.I. tract irritation, metallic taste, pain chest, etc. Pancreatitis is a usual feature. Serious side effects are bone marrow depression, shock and sudden unexplained death.

Pentamidine

It is a diamidine and is therapeutically used against Leishmania donovani, Pneumocystis carinii and Trypanosoma gambiense. It is toxic to parasitic cell but the exact mechanism of its action is not yet known. It damages pancreatic beta cells. Other side effects are acute hypotension, palpitations and dyspnoea.

Suramin

It is an organic urea compound used in the management of trypanosomiasis. Exact mechanism of its action is not known. It is also useful against adult form of Onchocerca volvulus. After treatment with suramin, trypanosomes lose their pathogenicity but do not die within 24 hours in vitro. It is always used intravenously. Binding to plasma protein is very strong and lasts for about 3 months after a single dose. However, it is not useful in encephalitis stage of trypanosomiasis as it cannot cross blood brain barrier. Under such circumstances, melarsoprol, an arsenical is useful. Suramin is nephrotoxic.

Chloroquine

Chloroquine (Fig. 8.2) is a 4-aminoquinoline derivative. It has powerful action against asexual erythrocytic form of Pl. vivax and Pl. falciperum. It is also effective against gametocytes of Pl. vivax, Pl. ovale and Pl. malariae but is ineffective against sporozoites, persistent tissue forms

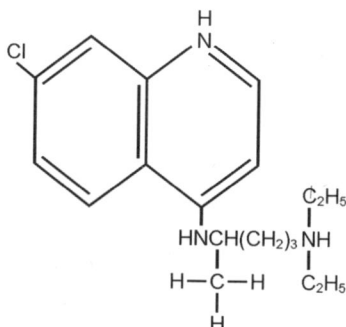

Fig.8.2. Chemical structure of chloroquine

and pre-erythrocytic forms. 4-Aminoquinolines possibly inhibit the incorporation of phosphate into RNA and DNA of malarial parasites and this may be its mechanism of schizonticidal effect. Chloroquine is safe during pregnancy.

On prolonged use, ocular complications like retinopathy, transient failure of accommodation, lental change, etc., may occur. Ototoxicity, convulsions, deranged ECG, various types of dermal allergic reactions, etc., are also seen during chloroquine therapy.

Apart from malaria, various parasitic disorders susceptible to chloroquine are taeniasis, giardiasis, amoebic hepatitis, Chinese liver fluke infestation, etc. It is also used in some systemic disorders like rheumatoid arthritis, discoid lupus erythematosus, infectious mononucleosis and in the management of acute lepra reaction.

Mebendazole

Mebendazole (Fig. 8.3) is a benzimidazole derivative. It is active against a large number of parasites like Ascaris lumbricoides, Ancylostoma duodenale, Necator americanus, Enterobius vermicularis, Trichuris trichiura, etc. It has also been found to be effective against hyatid cyst, larvae of Trichinella spiralis, etc. Exogenous glucose uptake required for existence of the parasite is blocked by mebendazole and ultimately the parasite is killed. The side effects are usually mild like nausea, vomiting, diarrhea, etc.

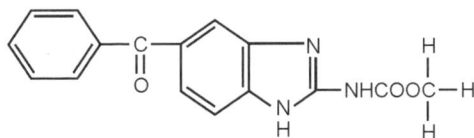

Fig. 8.3. Chemical structure of mebendazole

Albendazole

It is also a benzimidazole group of drug. The main advantage of this drug is that a single dose is usually required to eradicate most of the intestinal worms.

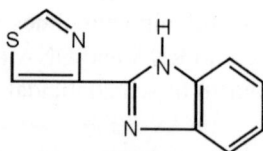

Fig. 8.4. Chemical structure of thiabendazole

Thiabendazole

It is a benzimidazole group of drug (Fig. 8.4) used mainly against cutaneous larva migrans and strongyloidiasis. It is also used against hookworms, round worms, dracontiasis, trichiniasis, trichuriasis, pinworms, etc. It acts as a blocker of essential metabolic pathways of worms. Milder side effects include gastrointestinal tract irritation and hypersensitive reactions. Serious side effects include liver and kidney damage.

Pyrantel Pamoate

It induces spastic paralysis in worms by acting as depolarizing neuromuscular blocking agent. Maximum effectiveness is seen in the cases of Ascaris lumbricoides and Enterobius vermicularis. Hookworms are also affected to some extent. Side effects are very mild like skin rash, gastrointestinal irritation, etc.

Levamisole

It (Fig. 8.5) is also a depolarizing neuromuscular blocking agent mainly active against Ascaris lumbricodes. It is also active (to a lesser extent) against hookworms. Side effects are mild.

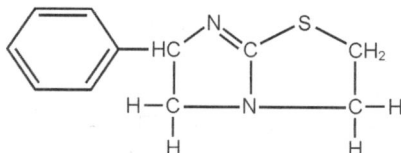

Fig. 8.5. Chemical structure of levamisole

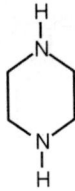

Fig. 8.6. Chemical structure of piperazine

Piperazine

Piperazine (Fig. 8.6) is a competitive neuromuscular blocking agent used mainly against Ascaris lumbricoides and Enterobius vermicularis. Citrate, hydrate, adipate and phosphate salts of piperazine are commonly used. It is a safe drug but sometimes neurotoxic effects are seen.

Diethylcarbamazine

It is a piperazine derivative (Fig. 8.7) and is active against the microfilariae of W. bancrofti, W. malayi and Loa loa. It helps to kill microfilaria by fixed reticuloendothelial cells of liver sinusoids and it also increases the cell mediated immunity of human beings. The drug is well tolerated but sometimes may produce hypersensitive reactions due to release of toxic materials from dead larvae or adult worms.

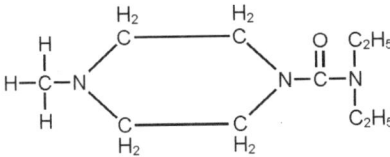

Fig. 8.7. Chemical structure of diethylcarbamazine

Ivermectin

It is a useful drug in the management of Onchocerca volvulus infestation. It causes paralysis of the worm by acting as GABA agonist and the worm is then scavenged by reticuloendothelial system. This drug is also useful in the management of scabies. Sometimes, toxins liberated by the dead microfilaria may induce severe uveitis leading to blindness.

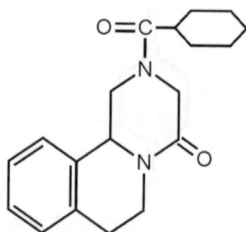

Fig. 8.8. Chemical structure of praziquantel

Praziquantel

Praziquantel (Fig. 8.8) is an important drug used in the treatment of intestinal, liver and lung flukes. It is also effective in Taenia solium infestation and has been used successfully in neurocysticercosis. It is a non-toxic drug, though a few cases may develop neurotoxicity. The drug kills the parasite by three ways:

- Restriction of glucose uptake.
- Violent muscular spasms.
- Vesicle formation on the surface.

Niclosamide

Niclosamide (Fig. 8.9) is an effective vermicidal drug used in the management of Taenia solium, Taenia saginata Diphyllobothrium latus, Hymenolepsis nana, etc. It mainly acts by suppression of anaerobic phosphorylation of ADP by mitochondria.

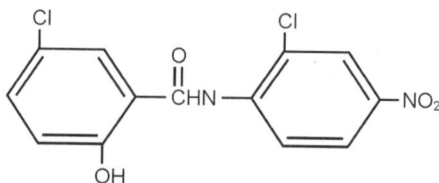

Fig. 8.9. Chemical structure of niclosamide

Bephenium Hydroxynaphthoate

It is a quaternary ammonium compound used mainly in the treatment of hookworm infestation. It causes contracture of the muscles of the parasite, so that they are expelled out by peristaltic movements.

Guidelines for Management of Some Parasitic Infestations in Relation to Eye

Protozoal Diseases

(1) **Amoebiasis.** Entamoeba histolytica can produce unilateral or bilateral choroiditis which may involve macula. The macular lesion may be haemorrhagic.

Treatment: Metronidazole-800 mg TDS (children 30-50 mg/kg/day) × 5 to 10 days.

(2) **Acanthamoeba Keratitis.** The condition is usually produced by A.castellani and A.polyphaga. No treatment is fully satisfactory. However, the commonly used treatment is as follows:

Neomycin + 0.1% propamidine isethionate (an aromatic diamidine) is used. 1 drop at ½ hourly intervals × 24 hours, then 1 hourly × 24 to 48 hours, then hourly during the waking hours, then every 2 hours; the course is continued for 2-3 months and ultimately maintenance dose is 1 drop thrice daily × 1 year. In case the treatment seems to be unsatisfactory, topical clotrimazole 1% to 2% may also be added to the above schedule.

(3) **Giardiasis.** G.lambia may cause uveitis. Any of the following drugs may be tried:

- Furazolidine – 100 mg 4 times a day × 7 days (children 1.25 mg/kg body weight, 4 times a day × 7 days.)
- Quinacrine – 100 mg thrice daily x 5 days (children 2 mg/kg/ day × 5 days)
- Metronidazole – 500 mg 4 times a day x 3 days (children 5 mg/kg thrice daily × 5 days).
- Tinidazole – 500 mg thrice daily × 5 days.
- Paromomycin – 25-30 mg/kg/day into 3 divided dose × 5 to 10 days. This is particularly useful during pregnancy.

(4) **Toxoplasmosis.** T. gondii causes posterior uveitis, necrotising retinochoroiditis, optic neuritis, papillitis, etc.

Treatment: the most popular and widely used treatment is Pyrimethamine 75 to 100 mg on 1st day, then 25 to 50 mg per day. Along with it, sulfadiazine 2 g on 1st day, then 1 g. qid × 4 to 6 wks may be given.

Other medicines used are clindamycin and atovaquone.

(5) **Leishmaniasis.**

- American Mucocutaneous Leishmaniasis: The causative organism is Leishmaina brasiliensis and it is transmitted by sandfly (genus Lutzomyia). In the eye, it causes blepharitis, keratitis, conjunctivitis and sometimes iridocyclitis. *Treatment*: Commonly used drug is sodium stibogluconate – 10 to 20 mg/kg/day – not exceeding a total dose of 600 mg I.M. or I.V. infusion × 15-25 days. The treatment may have to be repeated after 2 to 3 weeks. Ocular treatment with steroids, antibiotics and cycloplegics is concurrently done.

- Tropical sore (Cutaneous leishmaniasis): It is caused by Leishmania tropica and its vector is sandfly of genus Phlebotomus. A nodule occurs at the site of bite of fly which may ulcerate healing very slowly even without any treatment (by host immunity) taking about 1 year time. Usually, children are common victims. In the eye, the nodule is usually found in lids. However, the treatment of this condition is pentamidine isethionate – 4 mg/kg/day – I.M. or I.V. × 2 weeks.

- Kala-azar (Visceral leishmaniasis): It is caused by Leishmania donovani transmitted by sandfly (vector) of either genus previously mentioned. It is a systemic disease infecting R.E. system. Usually, spleen, liver and bone marrow are involved. The treatment is usually done with sodium stibogluconate or antimony meglumine.

(6) **Pneumocystis Carinii.** It usually affects AIDS patient in the form of pneumonia. Ocular involvement is rare and may occur in the form of choroidopathy comprising of numerous yellow-white foci. The treatment may be done by co-trimoxazole or pentamidine. Maintenance doses are often required. An example of line of treatment with pentamidine is 4 mg/kg/day – in 250 ml 5% dextrose solution – I.V. infusion for 1 hour × 2 to 3 weeks.

(7) **Malaria.** The causative organisms of malaria are Plasmodium vivax (benign tertian malaria), Pl malariae (quartan malaria), Pl falciparum (malignant tertian malaria) and Pl ovale (ovale malaria).

Involvement of eye is commonly seen with Plasmodium falciparum infection. Important eye lesions found in malaria are sub-conjunctival haemorrhage, keratitis, retinal haemorrhage, retinal detachment, optic neuritis, external ophthalmoplegia and orbital cellulitis. Basic line of treatment of falciparum and relapsing malaria is same. But in cases of relapsing malaria, to eradicate exoerythrocytic phase, radical curative drug therapy is also required. The treatment is as follows:

- Chloroquine – 600 mg to start with followed by 300 mg after 8 hours and then again 300 mg per day × 2 days.

In chloroquine-resistant or allergic cases:

- Pyrimethamine (25 mg) + sulphonamide (500 mg) – 3 tablets to be consumed in a single dose.

This cures the falciparum malaria. In case of resistant type of falciparum malariae, any one of the following treatments may be done:

- Quinine 300-600 mg TDS x 7 days either alone or along with pyrimethamine (75 mg) + sulphonamide (1500 mg) or along with tetracycline (250 mg Q.D.) or doxycycline (100 mg O.D).
- Mefloquine – 15 mg/kg (not exceeding a dose of 1 g) as single dose.
- Artesunate – 100 mg B.D. orally on 1st day and then 100 mg O.D. × 5 days. It may also be given I.M. or I.V. 120 mg on 1st day and then 60 mg/day × 4 days.
- Artemether – 80 mg BD on 1st day and then OD IM × 4 days.

In case of relapsing malaria (vivax / ovale) a radical curative drug which attacks exoerythrocytic phase (hypnozoites) is given just after the treatment with clinical curative drug (as has already been mentioned). Such drugs include Primaquine – 15 mg/day × 2 weeks.

(8) **Trypanosomiasis.** The most important is African trypanosomiasis (caused by Trypanosoma gambiense and T. rhodesiense, the vector being tsetse fly belonging to Glossina species) and American trypanomiasis (Chaga's disease caused by T.cruzi transmitted by reduviid bugs – mainly Triatoma infestans, Rhodnius prolixus and Panstrongylus megistus).

The main ocular lesions in African trypanosomiasis are edema of lids, interstitial keratitis, inflammation of uvea and optic neutitis. In the case of Chaga's disease, the main lesion produced is development of lid edema in one eye.

In African trypanosomiasis, pentamidine I.V. or I.M. in dosage 4 mg/kg/day is used × 10 days. If CNS is involved, melarsoprol 2 to

3.6 mg/kg/day in 3 divided doses I.V. is used (along with pentamidine) on 1st day, 8th day and 20th day. In Chaga's disease, nifurtimox is the drug of choice; the dose used is 8-10 mg/kg/day in 4 divided doses orally for 4 months.

Helminthic Diseases

Ocular helminthology can be divided into two broad groups:

I   Diseases caused by Phylum nemathelminths – class Nematoda.

II   Diseases caused by Phylum platyhelminths – class Trematoda and class Cestoda.

I. Class nematoda

(1) **Ascariasis**: It is caused by Ascaris lumbricoides. Various types of eye lesions include edema lids, chemosis of conjunctiva, keratoconjunctivitis, various forms of uveitis, papillitis, periphebitis, etc. These reactions may be direct hypersensitive reaction to Ascaris endotoxin or may be due to Type I allergic reaction. An effective treatment is achieved by oral mebendazole 100 mg BD x 3 days. This may be aided by surgical manipulation, e.g., removal of visible larva if any in A.C., vitreous or peripheral retina. In some cases, killing of larva is effective by laser treatment, if it is visible in retina. Supportive treatment includes local steroids, mydriatics and cold compress with plain water.

(2) **Enterobiasis**: The causative organism is Enterobius vermicularis and the eye lesion produced is mainly of antigen-antibody reaction type, being manifested by edema of the lids and keratoconjunctivitis. Out of the many drugs available for use, mebendazole is most popular and is used orally as a single dose, 100 mg. Supportive treatments include local steroid therapy, cold compress, antihitaminics, etc.

(3) **Ankylostomiasis**: The most important causative organisms of this group are Ankylostoma duodenale and Necator americanus. The eyes may be affected either by severe anaemia or by direct damage by larvae. Direct damage by larvae is manifested by cataract formation, retinopathies (haemorrhagic or exudative type), optic neuritis, etc. Another variant is diffuse unilateral subacute neuroretinitis (DUSN) manifested by various types of retinitis, optic neuritis, vitritis, degenerative changes in retinal pigment epithelial layer, etc. Sometimes,

larva can be observed moving around in subretinal space. DUSN can be caused by various other ocular migrating larvae also (e.g. larvae of Alaria species, Ankylostona caninum, Toxocara group, Baylisascaris procyonis, etc.). Therapeutic portions consist of (i) management of anaemia and (ii) deworming.

Anaemia needs treatment with iron, and other nutritive substances. The most popular deworming agent is pyrantel pamoate used as a single dose 10 mg/kg/day ×1-3 days. Pyrantel kills co-existing ascaris also (if present). For arresting visual damage, steroid therapy is also needed. DUSN is best managed by laser therapy.

(4) **Loasis**: The causative organism is Loa loa. Intermediate host is a blood sucking fly of species Chrysops. The common habitat of this worm is subcutaneous tissue near eye; hence, it is popularly known as eye worm. The worm produces swelling called calabar swelling, which can be found anywhere in the body but most commonly around the eyes. The lesions produced usually are edema of lids and, sometimes, exophthalmos. Sometimes, microfilaria is seen below the conjunctiva. The most widely accepted treatment is with diethylcarbamazine citrate, 50 mg on first day, increasing the dose to 50 mg t.d on second day, 100 mg t.d on third day and then a maintenance dose 2 to 3 mg/kg/t.d up to third week. A repetition of treatment may be required again. Subconjunctival filaria is removed surgically. Along with it, a supportive treatment with steroids, antihistaminics and antipyretics may be needed. It is also important to know a prophylactic treatment, particularly for tourists traveling in endemic areas: a course of diethylcarbamazine citrate, 100 mg to be taken twice in a month or 5 mg/kg/day for 3 days in a month.

(5) **Wuchereriasis**: It is caused by Wuchereria bancrofti and W.malayi. The intermediate host is female Culex fatigans. Eye involvement is rare, but sometimes elephantiasis of lids and retinal haemorrhage have been reported. The recommended treatment is Ivermectin – 150 microgram/kg – single dose to be taken once every 3 months. 2 to 4 such courses may be needed. However, diethylcarbamazine citrate therapy is needed to get rid of adult worms.

(6) **Onchocerciasis**: The causative organism is Onchocerca volvulus in Africa and O. caecutiens in middle and South America. Their life span is about 15 years. The intermediate host is a female black fly (which sucks blood) belonging to the species Simulium damnosum

(most common), which resides and breeds near fast flowing rivers (e.g. Volta river vally of Africa). Hence, in the endemic areas, this disease is also known as 'river-blindness'. The disease may also be carried to fetus through transplacental circulation (although rare). There is formation of helminthomas on facial and eyelid skin. Ocular involvement includes conjunctivitis, keratitis, uveitis, optic neuritis, etc. These reactions are believed to be due to antigen-antibody reaction – the protein component coming from dead worms. Sometimes, motile microfilaria can be observed in cornea, anterior chamber, vitreous cavity and even on retina.

The most modern treatment is with ivermectin which cannot kill the adult worm but makes it less fertile. The treatment consists of 150 to 200 microgram ivermectin per kg body weight once every 12 months for a period of 12 to 15 years. The old treatment with diethylcarbamazine citrate followed by suramin therapy is practically out of date, as it creates a lot of problems by inducing antigen-antibody reaction. A newer addition in the management of this disease is amocarazine, which is an adult worm killer plus microfilaricide, but it has hepatic and neurological side effects. Its dose is 3 mg/kg/BD × 3 days orally.

(7) **Dracunculosis**: The causative organism is guineaworm – Dracunculus medinensis -- and the intermediate host is Cyclops. Cases have been reported (although few) of adult worms causing proptosis and also moving in subconjunctival tissue space and intraocular space. Typical traditional treatment is to allow the worm to come out comfortably (winding round a stick and putting water to prevent its dehydration), because if the worm is killed there may be violent allergic and/ or pyogenic inflammation. Only option is to use some drugs to facilitate its exit. For this purpose, metronidazole 250 mg t.d. × 10 days and thiabendazole 25 mg/kg BD × 2 to 3 days are used. Niridazole is also effective, 25 mg/ kg/day in divided doses × 7 days.

(8) **Toxocariasis**: It is caused by Toxocara canis (normal parasite of dog) or Toxocara catis (normal parasite of cat). Human infection is purely accidental and in no way related to normal life cycle of worm. Ocular lesions caused by it are formation of retinal granuloma, endophthalmitis, uveitis, traction detachment of retina, etc.

' Treatment of ocular complications is done by cryotherapy, photocoagulation, vitreous surgery, steroid therapy, etc. Orally, as an anthelmintic, thiabendazole 25-50 mg/kg per day in two divided doses × 7-10 days is used. The treatment may have to be repeated once or twice again.

(9) **Gnathostomiasis**: Causative organism is Gnathostoma spinigerum or G. hispidum. The normal hosts are dog, cat and wild animals like tiger. Intermediate host is Cyclops which is eaten up by fishes, frogs, snakes. When a man eats undercooked meat of these animals (e.g. fish), he gets infected but that marks the biological end of the life of parasite. There is usually nodule formation or abscess formation mainly on skin, but involvement of CNS or eyes has also been reported.

If possible, the parasite should be removed surgically. Common anthelmintic drug used is albendazole 400 mg BD × 21 days.

(10) **Baylisascariasis**: The causative organism is Baylisascaris procyonis and the natural host is raccoons. Human beings are accidentally infected. The most important eye lesion produced by the larvae is DUSN.

Medical therapy is unsatisfactory. However, thiabendazole, 22 mg/kg BD × 2-4 days, has been tried. Laser treatment can also be tried in case the larvae are visible in ocular tissues.

(11) **Angiostrongyliasis**: The causative organism is Angiostrongylus cantonensis, which comes from various rodents including rat. The intermediate hosts are fish, crab, prawn, snails, etc. Humans get accidentally infected by consuming undercooked preparation of the above mentioned intermediate hosts. Ocular lesions are rare but there may be retinal detachment, optic neuritis and direct invasion of intravitreal and subretinal space by larvae. Meningoencephalitis is the main disease caused by the parasite.

Surgical removal should be attempted in case the worm is visible. Mebendazole 100 mg BD × 5 days has been tried with satisfactory results.

(12) **Trichinosis**: The causative organism is Trichinella spiralis. It has no intermediate host. Animal reservoirs include various carnivores, swine, rats, etc. Humans usually get infected by undercooked pork. The parasite after passing through different phases passes to a striated muscle. Extraocular muscles are also susceptible for their shelter. Ultimately, the matured worm is encapsulated by the host. After an initial period of vomiting and diarrhoea, there are enteric fever-like features. Later on, there is edema of the extraocular muscle concerned.

Various features like subconjunctival haemorrhage, retinal haemorrhage and exudative retinitis have been reported. Local ocular treatment with steroids, cycloplegics may be required. Drug therapy is not satisfactory. During intestinal phase (very difficult to identify), thiabendazole-25 mg/kg/day × 5 days may be tried. During muscle invasion phase, mebendazole 200-400 mg t.d. × 3 days followed by 400-500 mg t.d. × 10 days has been found to be effective to some extent.

(13) **Dirofilariasis**: The causative organisms are Dirofilaria immitis (host-dog), Dirofilaria repens (hosts-dogs and cats) and D. tennius (host-raccoons). Mosquito is the vector which transmits the larvae to human beings. But, as the environment in human body is not satisfactory for growth of the adult worm in the usual manner, after maturing to some extent, the worm gets encapsulated and dies either within cardio-pulmonary system or subcutaneous tissue.

Ocular lesions produced by the worms are exophthalmos (due to orbital cyst formation), infiltration in AC, vitreous cavity, subconjunctival space, etc. The usual treatment is diethylcarbamazine citrate and the dose is same as for Loa Loa infestation (see earlier text).

(14) **Thelaziasis**: The causative organism is a nematode belonging to genus Thelazia. The normal habitats of adult worms are conjunctival sac and lacrimal sac. Flies act as both vector and intermediate host transmitting the disease to other animals and also to human beings.

Ocular involvement is restricted to conjunctival sac and some time AC. Inflammation of conjunctival sac is a common feature. Visible worm (most commonly found in conjunctival fornices) should always be removed mechanically. The medicinal treatment is diethylcarbamazine citrate, 50 mg TD × 14 days.

II. Phylum Platyhelminths, class trematoda (flukes)

(1) **Lung fluke infestation (Paragonimiasis)**: The causative organism is Paragonimus westermani. Life cycle of all flukes is quite complicated. Man is the definitive host and intermediate hosts are snails and crustaceans. The adult worm lives in the lungs of human beings with an average life span of approximately 10 years. Ocular lesions may be due to involvement of CNS or due to direct attack on eye (producing violent uveitis).

The parasite should be removed surgically from the eye. Systemic therapy is usually done with praziquantel, 25 mg/kg t.d × 3 days. Alternatively, treatment is done with bithionol, 30-50 mg/kg on alternate days; the treatment is to be done for 10-15 days.

(2) Blood fluke infestation (Schistosomiasis, Bilharziasis): The causative organisms are Schistosoma haematobium, S. mansoni, S. japonicum and S. mekongi. S. haematobium may reside in dogs, cats, deer, cattle and humans, but others utilize only human beings as the definitive host. The intermediate hosts are snails. Sexually matured worms live in pairs in veins usually at vesical or pelvic venous piexus. Ocular involvement has been reported. There may be granuloma formation (in case they reside at venous channel near eyeball) in uvea, lacrimal sac, or even conjunctiva. Granulomas, if approachable, should be surgically removed. Medical treatment is usually done with praziquantel 40 mg/kg to be given on a day in two divided doses in the case of S. haematobium and mansoni. In the case of S. Japonioum and S. mekongi, 60 mg/kg is to be given on a day in 3 divided doses. After this, a course of niridazole 12.5 mg/kg BD x 7 days is advocated.

(3) Trematodes belonging to Alaria species: Sometimes the mesocercariae type of larve of Alaria species may infect man and produce ocular lesions DUSN.

Surgical procedures (in case the larva is visible) should be attempted. Medical treatment with albendazole or praziquantel along with steroids (if required) may be helpful.

II. Phylum Platyhelminths, class cestoda (tape worms)

(1) Cysticercosis: The causative organisms are Taenia solium and T. saginata. Man is the definitive host. In the case of T. solium, pig is usually the intermediate host, and in the case of T. saginata, cattle are the most important intermediate hosts. In the body of pig, larval stage cysticerous cellulosae is formed. Accidentally, man can also develop cysticercus cellulosae. However, in the case of T. saginata, the larval stage is formed in the body of cattle, called cysticercus bovis. Man never gets this larval form of disease because the larvae cannot penetrate human mucosa.

Cysticercus cellulosae have been found to occur in vitreous chamber, AC, under conjunctiva and retina and even in orbit. Surgical removal of cysticercus is the treatment of choice. Medical treatment in case of ocular cysticercosis is done by metrifonate 75 mg/kg/day x 5 days; it may be repeated after two weeks again.

For extraocular disease, treatment is Albendazole 15 mg/kg/day in divided doses 8 days. Alternatively, praziquantel 50 mg/kg/day in three divided doses × 15 days may be given.

(2) **Echinococcosis**: The name of the causative organism is Echinococcus granulosus (formerly called Taenia echinococcus). Dog is the definitive host and sheep is the intermediate host. Humans may sometimes be infected acting as the intermediate hosts. The disease caused in humans is called hydatid disease. Mainly, these cysts are formed in liver and lungs but other organs like CNS, kidney, bones, spleen, etc., may be involved. If eye is involved there may be orbital cyst giving rise to exophthalmos. Sometimes, intraocular cysts and cysts in the lids are also found. Classically, the cysts are removed surgically. But in the cases of large cysts, there is a chance of rupture and there may be dissemination of larvae to surrounding tissues. So, initially the cyst is punctured and material aspirated. Then the cyst is inflated with alcohol (70%), sodium chloride (20%), formaldehyde (1%), cetrimide (5%) and silver nitrate (0.5%) or sodium hypochlorite (3.75%). This mixture is allowed to stay in the cyst for 5 min and then the chemicals are aspirated. Next the cyst wall is excised. Medical treatment of echinococcosis consists of Mebendazole, 50 mg/kg/day in 3 divided doses x 1 month. The course needs a repetition after 3 to 6 months. Alternatively, treatment consists of albendazole 800 mg/ day in 4 divided doses x 28 days. It needs 3 such courses with two weeks' intervals.

(3) **Coenurosis**: The causative organism is a tapeworm belonging to genus Multiceps. Definitive host is usually dog and intermediate host is sheep. Humans may get accidentally infected and there is formation of cyst called coenurus in brain, subcutaneous tissue, muscles and eyes. In eye, the cyst may form in subconjunctival tissue, A.C., vitreous, choroid, retina, etc. The coenurus should be removed surgically through pars plana route when it is in posterior portion of globe. Medical treatment is praziquantel, 25 to 50 mg/ kg/ day × 14 days.

(4) **Sparganosis**: The causative organism identified so far is spirometra cestodes. Its life cycle is complicated. The definitive host is usually dog or cat. Intermediate hosts are many in different stages of the life

cycle of larva. They include cyclops, amphibians, reptiles, etc. Humans may be accidentally infected through intermediate hosts. When infected, nodules develop containing larvae called sparganum. Such nodules are found in peritoneum, brain, abdominal viscera and eyes. When eye is involved, the features of SOL are seen. The treatment is essentially surgical. Medical treatment of some value is with neoarsphenamine, 300 to 450 mg 2 to 6 times a day every 4 to 5 days.

Ectoparasite Induced Diseases

(1) **Diseases caused by tick**: Tick may cause various diseases like borreliosis. It is caused by Borrelia burgdorferi, which is a spirochete and may produce eye lesions like keratoconjunctivitis, uveitis and retinitis, and neurological involvement. The present day treatment is to remove the ticks within 24 hours.

(2) **Diseases caused by louse**: The cilia are infested mainly by crab louse Phthirus pubis. Mainly, severe blepharitis and haemorrhagic crusts are seen to be attached to the skin at lid margin. The best way of treatment is removal by forceps and epilating the lash where nits are attached. However, in severe cases lashes are cut and then the lid margin is painted with 1% silver nitrate solution. Thereafter, physostigmime ointment is applied as it paralyses the muscular system of parasite. However, the treatment has to be continued for two weeks. A currently used medicine is 1% watery shampoo of malathion, which is a cholinersterase inhibitor, and needs 1 to 2 applications. Shampoo is to be applied by a cotton swab and has to be washed off completely after 5 minutes. A through treatment of the whole body and all members of the family should to be done to prevent relapses.

(3) **Ophthalmomyiasis**: It is a condition where the infestation occurs by larvae of flies. Superficial infestation causing conjunctivitis may occur due to larvae of Oestrus ovis and Rhinoestrus purpureus. First of all, one should try to remove the maggots mechanically followed by application of cholinesterase inhibitor to paralyze the worm. Steroids and antibiotics may be needed to combat inflammation and sepsis. This type of infestation is also called external ophthalmomyiasis.

In some cases, internal penetration of larvae can occur, causing endophthalmitis. The species of flies of this category are Hypoderma bovis, Wohlfahrtia magnifica, Oestrus ovis, etc. This clinical condition produced is also called internal ophthalmomyiasis. Surgical removal is the only treatment, unless a secondary infection supervenes.

There is a fly, Hypoderma bovis, whose maggots can migrate into deep orbital structure, causing inflammation and producing exophthalmos. It is a frustrating condition. Treatment is unsatisfactory. However, antibiotics, steroids, surgical removal, etc., are advocated.

Another addition to this series is larva of Dermatobia hominis which can reside underneath skin forming a swelling. Skin of eyelid may be affected. Here again, the larva has to be surgically removed aided by local anaesthetic and physostigmine ointment.

(4) Diseases caused by mite: Mites causing infestation of hair follicles and Meibomian glands of lid belong to genus Demodex (D. folliculorum and D. brevis). Common features are itching and burning sensation of lid margins.

The usual treatment is repeated application of ether at lid margin by a cotton swab stick. An ointment containing a mixture of 1% yellow oxide of mercury plus 2% white mercury precipitate is also effective. Other useful drugs are potassium polysulfide ointment and erythromycin ointment.

CHAPTER 9

Adrenocortical Steroids

Hormones Secreted by Adrenal Gland

Adrenal gland is one of the important endocrine glands of human body. It has two parts: cortex and medulla. The hormones secreted from the adrenal cortex are glucocorticoids, mineralocorticoids and sex corticoids (Fig. 9.1).

(a) *Glucocorticoids*: They are synthesized from zona fasciculata (mainly) and from zona reticularis, parts of adrenal gland.

(b) *Mineralocorticoids*: They are synthesized and secreted from zona glomerulosa part of adrenal gland.

(c) *Sex corticoids*: They are synthesized and secreted from zona reticularis part of adrenal cortex.

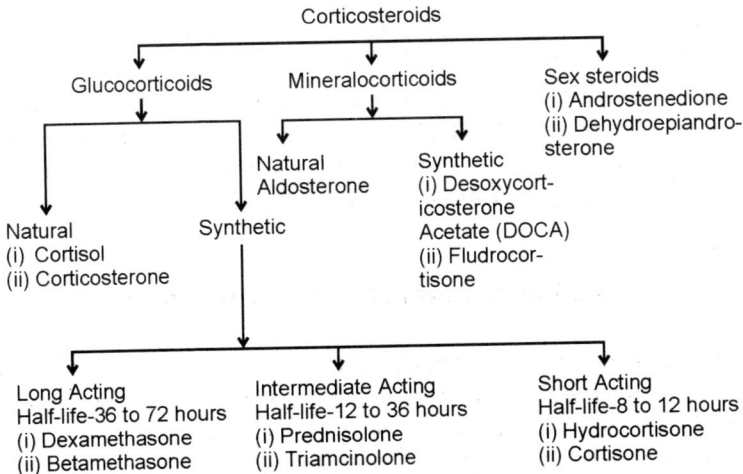

Corticosteroids

Glucocorticoids — Mineralocorticoids — Sex steroids
(i) Androstenedione
(ii) Dehydroepiandro-
sterone

Natural Aldosterone — Synthetic
(i) Desoxycort-
icosterone
Acetate (DOCA)
(ii) Fludrocor-
tisone

Natural — Synthetic
(i) Cortisol
(ii) Corticosterone

Long Acting
Half-life-36 to 72 hours
(i) Dexamethasone
(ii) Betamethasone

Intermediate Acting
Half-life-12 to 36 hours
(i) Prednisolone
(ii) Triamcinolone

Short Acting
Half-life-8 to 12 hours
(i) Hydrocortisone
(ii) Cortisone

Fig. 9.1. A diagram illustrating classification of corticosteroids

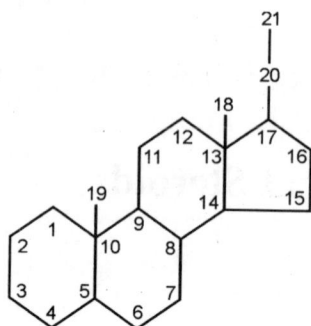

Fig. 9.2. Basic chemical structure of CPP ring

These hormones are steroid hormone, of which cholesterol molecule is the basic pharmacological structure. All of them contain a cyclopentanoperhydro-phenanthrene (CPP) ring (Fig. 9.2).

These hormones are lipid-soluble and thus directly enter inside the cell and act directly on intra-nuclear receptors. They elicit their function by stimulating/inhibiting some specific protein synthesis.

Regulation of Corticosteroid Secretion (Fig. 9.3)

Adrenocorticotrophic hormone (ACTH), secreted from anterior pituitary is responsible for the growth and development of adrenal cortex and the release of the hormones. Glucocorticoids and minerelocorticoids thus released inhibit further ACTH secretion (feedback inhibition).

Corticotrophin releasing factor (CRF) released from hypothalamus controls secretion of ACTH. It is secreted when adrenaline is released from adrenal medulla under stress situations. Normally, CRF is released in pulsatile manner, so also is ACTH.

Action of Adrenal Cortex Hormones

Though all corticosteroids have some distinct action on human body, due to structural similarity they overlap to some extent. For example, corticosteroids can stimulate Na^+ re-absorption and K^+ and H^+ excretion from distal convoluted tubule of nephron of kidney though it is major action of mineralocorticoids.

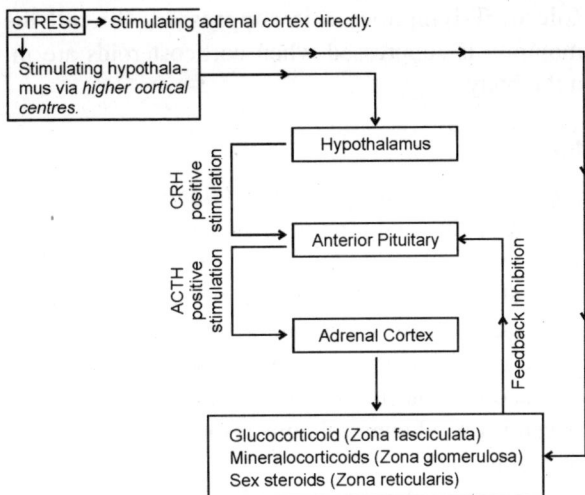

Fig. 9.3. Diagram illustrating regulation of corticosteroid secretion

Action of Glucocorticoids on Metabolism

(a) *Carbohydrate metabolism*: Glucocorticoids cause hyperglycaemia by stimulating glycogenolysis, neoglucogenesis and glycogenesis in liver.

(b) *Protein and fat metabolism*: Mainly, catabolic effect is observed on protein metabolism. There is muscle wasting, thinning of bone and skin. The broken down protein is used for neoglucogenesis. There is increased formation of urea and excretion of uric acid. The main action on fat metabolism is lipolysis. There is a peculiar type of distribution of fat – mobilization from periphery and accumulation at neck, face and supraclavicular regions giving rise to characteristic moon face, buffalo hump and fish mouth.

(c) *Immunological mechanism*: Glucocorticoids inhibit all types of inflammatory and allergic (hypersensitivity) mechanisms.

- Reduce capillary permeability.
- Inhibit phagocytosis.
- Prevent migration of phagocytic cells.
- Inhibit formation of inflammatory mediators like prostaglandin and leukotrienes.

- Role of T-lymphocyte is suppressed. So cell mediated immunity is suppressed when corticosteroids are in excess in the body.

Other actions

(a) *Effect on cardiovascular system*: Glucocorticoids maintain myocardial contractility and tone of arterioles.

(b) *Effect on musculoskeletal system*: Both hypercorticism and hypocorticism affect the skeletal muscle adversely. When in excess, glucocorticoid causes hypokalemia and when deficient it reduces blood flow leading to lack of oxygen supply to muscle.

Excess glucocorticoid reduces bone density (decreased osteoid) and hypocalcemia by reducing calcium absorption and increased renal calcium excretion.

(c) *Effect on gastrointestinal system*: Glucocorticoids increase acid and pepsin secretion.

(d) *Effect on central nervous system*: Excess glucocorticoid causes insomnia, anxiety whereas reduced level causes apathy, depression, etc.

(e) *Effect on haematological system*: Glucocorticoids raise neutrophil and RBC numbers, but lymphocyte, eosinophil and basophil numbers fall.

Action of Minerelocorticoids

Mineralocorticoid acts on distal convoluted tubule of nephron of kidney to re-absorb Na^+ at the cost of K^+ and H^+ excretion. Deficiency may ultimately lead to circulatory collapse, while excessive mineralocorticoid activity may cause fluid retention and hypertension.

Ophthalmic Use of Corticosteroids

Ophthalmic Indications

- Conjunctival diseases: (i) Vernal conjunctivitis, (ii) Phlyctenulosis
- Scleral diseases: (i) Episcleritis, (ii) Scleritis
- Uveitis

- Prophylactic use against proliferative vitreoretinopathy
- Retrobulbar neuritis
- To prevent rejection of corneal graft
- Miscellaneous conditions: (i) Harada's disease, (ii) Grave's orbitopathy, (iii) Pseudotumour of orbit and (iv) Behcet's disease

Non-ophthalmic Indications of Corticosteroids

Other than ophthalmic indications, corticosteroids are used in various types of adrenal insufficiency (primary, secondary, etc.), anaphylactic shock, various types of vasculitis, status asthmaticus, rheumatic fever, cerebral edema, as chemotherapeutic agents in different hematological malignancies and many other medical disorders.

Routes of Administration of Corticosteroids in Eye

Topical

Commonly used steroids applied as eye drops or ointments are dexamethasone, betamethasone, hydrocortisone, prednisolone, fluorometholone, medroxy progesterone and some newer drugs like Loteprednol etabonate and rimexolone. Out of these, medroxyprogesteron has weak anti-inflammatory property, but significant anti collagenase activity and, hence, it is very useful in alkali burns of cornea.

Loteprednol Etabonate. It possesses no systemic side effects as it is quickly inactivated by cellular esterase, but it may cause a slight rise in intraocular pressure.

Rimexolone. It has a very insignificant role in raising intraocular tension, but is a very potent (like prednisolone) anti-inflammatory agent.

Subconjunctival injection

Though this route is used to increase anterior chamber concentration of steroid, it is found that desired concentration is not reached. On the other hand, more effective concentration can be achieved by frequent drop applications.

Retrobulbar and periocular route

Crystalline suspensions are used to sustain its effects for 4-8 weeks. Considerable concentrations are achieved in vitreous, optic nerve and uveal tract without any significant systemic effect. But steroid induced glaucoma may develop. It is also not suitable for scleritis.

Intra-vitreal route

It is used in endophthalmitis and in prophylaxis of proliferative vitreo retinopathy.

Systemic route

It is generally indicated in those ocular conditions which are actually a part of systemic autoimmune disorders as mentioned earlier. Preparation used is preferably prednisolone (t1/2 – 12-36 hours) given orally at breakfast table (about 9.00 a.m.). Divided dosage is usually avoided to keep pituitary hypothalamus adrenal axis intact.

A more recent addition is pulse steroid therapy where methyl prednisolone 1 g I.V. thrice per week is given. Trial to this treatment has been given in optic neuritis, various types of uveitis not responding to usual treatment and many other conditions where usual type of treatment has been found to be of no value. When using systematically for more than 2 weeks, steroids should be tapered off to prevent flaring up of the disease concerned and to allow pituatry adrenal axis to resume its function. When treatment period is 3-6 weeks, gradual tapering is the rule. Use of systemic steroid for more than 6 weeks should be avoided as there may be complete suppression of adrenal cortex. But in the case of corneal transplantation, prophylaxis in suspected giant cell arteritis and in pulse therapy in traumatic optic neuropathy tapering is not required.

Preparations

Following are the commonly used preparations.

Topical preparations

- Betamethasone sodium phosphate solution, 0.1%.
- Hydrocortisone acetate solution, 1% and ointment, 2.5%.

- Prednisolone acetate suspension, 0.125%, 1%, 0.12%.
- Prednisolone sodium phosphase solution, 0.125%, 1.00%, 0.5%.
- Dexamethasone alcohol suspension, 0.1%.
- Dexamethasone sodium phosphate solution and ointment 0.05%, 0.1%.
- Fluorometholone alcohol ointment, 0.1% and suspensions, 0.1% and 0.25%.
- Medroxyprogesterone, 1% eye drop.
- Lotoprednol elabonate, 0.5% suspension.
- Rimexolone, 1% suspension.

Systemic preparations

- Hydrocortisone sodium succinate injection; vial contains 100 mg hydrocortisone – 1.M./1.V.
- Prednisolone tabs 5, 10, 20 and 40 mg.
- Methylprednisolone injection I.M. or I.V., available as 40 mg/ml.
- Dexamethasone tabs 0.5 mg and inj. 4 mg/ml in 2 ml vial.
- Betamethasone tabs 0.5 mg and inj. 4 mg/ml.
- Triamcinolone tablets, 4 mg and inj. 10 mg/ml – 1 ml injection.

Doses of commonly used systemic steroids

- Prednisolone 5 to 60 mg per day orally.
- Dexamethasone 0.5 to 5 mg per day orally. Can also be used 4-20 mg per day as I.M. inj. or I.V. infusion.
- Betamethasone – 0.5 to 5 mg per day orally. Can also be used 4-20 mg per day I.M. or I.V.
- Triamcinolone – 4 to 32 mg per day orally. Can also be used 5 to 40 mg per day I.M.

Contraindications of Steroid Application

Steroid application is contraindicated in the following cases:
- Hypertension
- Diabetes mellitus

- Peptic ulcer
- Osteoporosis
- Tuberculosis
- Herpes simplex keratitis
- Psychiatric problem
- Pregnancy
- Congestive cardiac failure
- Renal failure
- Epilepsy

Drug Interactions

Some agents inhibit corticosteroid synthesis like metyrapone, ketoconazole, aminoglutethimide, etc. Spironolactone acts as aldosterone receptor antagonist.

INH, ketoconazole, cyclosporin, erythromycin, etc., reduce metabolic clearance along with reduction of free fraction by increasing amount of corticosteroid binding protein (CBP). Cholestyramine decreases corticosteroid absorption. Barbiturate, rifampicin, carbamazepine phenytoin, etc., increase metabolism of corticosteroid by enzyme induction. These drug interactions are important, and dose adjustment is required for their concurrent administration.

Ocular Side Effects of Steroids

Ocular side effects of steroids are:
- Cataract
- Glaucoma
- Miscellaneous, like (i) delay in corneal wound healing (due to retardation in collagen synthesis), (ii) susceptibility to infection (due to immunosuppression), (iii) diffuse retinal pigment epitheliopathy and (iv) pseudotumour cerebri.

Steroid Responders

It has been observed statistically that 30% of general population show an increase in IOP 6-15 mm Hg and 4-5% show increase in IOP> 15 mm Hg. This rise may occur 2-3 weeks after application of drug, but it may be delayed by as much as 4-6 months. Such people are called steroid responders. Suggested mechanisms for such rise in IOP following topical steroid application are:

- Deposition of mucopolysaccharides in trabecular meshwork.
- Decrease in the permeability of outflow channels.
- A tightening effect in lysosomal membrane.
- An excessive formation of aqueous humour.
- Deposition of glycoseaminoglycans at trabecular meshwork.
- Reduction in synthesis of prostaglandins, which regulate aqueous humour outflow.

Systemic Side Effects of Steroids

Systemic side effects of steroids are:

- G.I. Tract – peptic ulcer, intestinal perforation, pancreatitis, etc.
- Immunity – increased infection, delayed wound healing.
- CVS – hypertension.
- CNS – psychosis, benign intra cranial hypertension.
- Renal system – salt and water retention, hyperkalemic acidosis.
- Musculoskeletal system – myopathy, osteoporosis.
- Endocrine system – hyperglycaemia, suppression of pituitary adrenal axis.
- Others – Cushing's syndrome, slowing of growth rate in children, atrophy of subcutaneous tissue fat, hirsutism, baldness, thromboembolic disorders.

CHAPTER 10

Non-steroidal Anti-inflammatory Drugs (NSAIDs)

These drugs are frequently used in various types of ocular inflammatory disorders as well as in some systemic inflammatory conditions like systemic lupus erythematosus, rheumatoid arthritis and psoriatic arthritis, which may cause ophthalmic complications.

Though corticosteroids are more powerful anti-inflammatory agents, their usage over a long period of time is not desirable due to adverse side effects.

Eicosanoids

Prostaglandins, thromboxanes and leukotrienes are all derivatives of 20-carbon atom containing compounds, eicosa acids (trienoic, tetraenoic, pentaenoic acids), and so they are called eicosanoids as a group. Any type of stimulus (mechanical, chemical, immunological, etc) may activate hydrolases (e.g. phospholipase A) which release arachidonic acid from membrane phospholipid.

Arachidonic acid thus formed may undergo either cyclo-oxygenase (COX) pathway giving rise to ecosanoids with ring structures like prostaglandins, thromboxanes, prostacycline, etc., or alternatively undergo lipooxygenase pathway (LOX) giving rise to open chain compounds like leukotrienes.

Lungs and spleen are two main organs which can produce all derivatives of cyclooxygenase pathway. Platelets are mainly concerned with synthesis of thromboxane TXA2 which rapidly gets converted into TXB2; prostacycline is mainly produced by vessel wall but this soon gets converted into 6-keto PGF1 alpha.

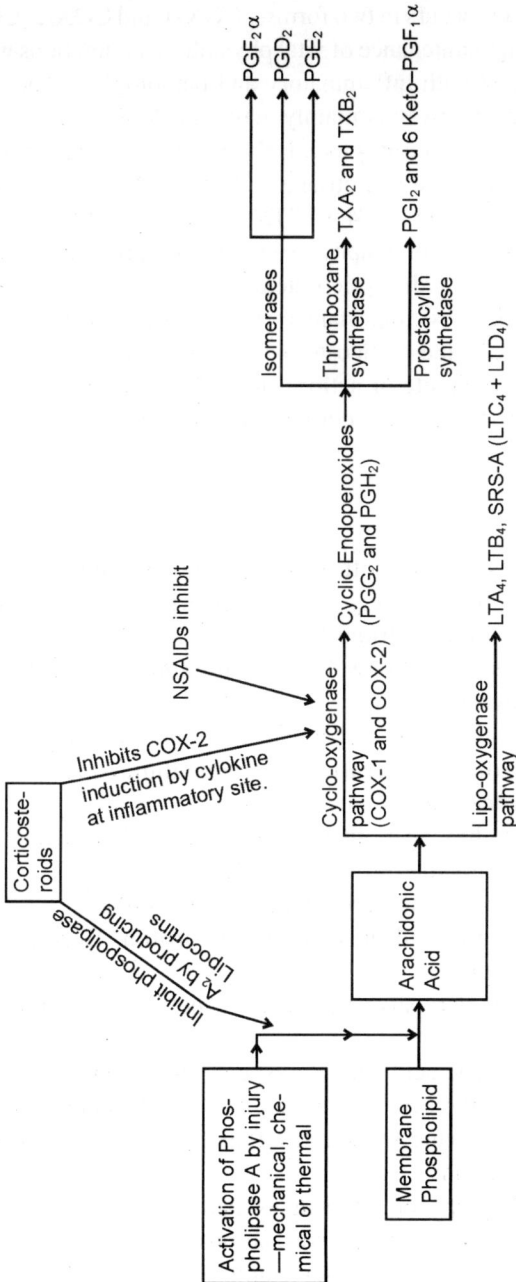

Fig. 10.1. A diagram illustrating sites of action of NSAIDs and corticosteroids during inflammatory process

Cyclooxygenase occurs in two forms – COX-1 and COX-2. COX-1 is concerned with maintenance of vital physiological functions while COX-2 is concerned with inflammatory and pathological processes. Lipooxygenase pathway is mainly active in WBC, platelets and lungs. As has already been discussed, the most important products produced in this series are leukotrienes. Of these, LTB4 is a potent chemotactic substance and LTC4 + LTD4 together constitute SRS-A (slow reacting substance of anaphylaxis). Another product produced by LOX is 12 HETE (hydroxyeicosatetraenoic acid). Generation of prostaglandin is the most important factor during an inflammatory process. Both NSAID and corticosteroid can block the generation of prostaglandin, but their site of action varies. Fig 10.1 illustrates the sites of action of NSAIDs and corticosteroids during inflammatory process.

Classification

(a) Substances having both powerful anti-inflammatory and analgesic properties: e.g., salicylates (which include sodium salicylate, aspirin, diflunisal, etc.)

(b) Substances having powerful anti-inflammatory action but weak analgesic action:

   (i) Indole derivatives: indomethacin, sulindac, etc.

   (ii) Pyrazolone derivatives: oxyphenbutazone, phenyl-butazone, etc.

(c) Substances having both moderate anti-inflammatory and analgesic properties:

   (i) Pyrrolo-pyrrole derivatives, e.g., ketorolac.

   (ii) Propionic acid derivatives: ibuprofen, flurbiprofen, naproxen, etc.

   (iii) Oxicam derivatives: piroxicam, meloxicam, tenoxicam, etc.

   (iv) Aryl acetic acid derivatives, e.g., diclofenac.

   (v) Anthranilic acid derivatives, e.g., Mephenamic acid.

(d) Substances having weak anti-inflammatory action but good analgesic action:

   (i) Para-aminophenol derivatives: paracetamol.

   (ii) Benzoxazocine derivatives: nefopam.

   (iii) Pyrazolone derivatives: metamizole

(e) Miscellaneous agents mainly active against Cox-2: Nimesulide, Celecoxib, Rofecoxib, Valdecoxib, etc.

Mechanism of Action

All NSAIDs inhibit cyclooxygenase pathway leading to depression in synthesis and release of prostaglandins; COX inhibition is irreversible by aspirin group (by acetylation process). Other drugs like propionic acid derivatives and oxicams act by competitive inhibition.

During an inflammatory process, the lysosomal membranes of polymorphs release enzymes. Indomethacin group of drugs prevent such release of enzymes by inhibition of phosphodiesterase leading to increased concentration of cyclic AMP, which in turn stabilizes the lysosomal membrane (of polymorphs).

Release of lymphokines from activated T-lymphocytes is also prevented by aspirin group. Similarly, diclofenac and indomethacin suppress release of leukotrienes from WBC.

All NSAIDs suppress free radicals and superoxides.

Important Pharmacological Action of NSAIDs

* *Anti-inflammatory action*: NSAID decreases the level of vasodilator substances like PGE2 and PGI2 as a result of which inflammatory edema is prevented.
* *Antipyretic action*: During an inflammatory process, pyrogen substances like interleukin – 1, etc., are formed. These substances produce chemical mediator like PGE2 which upsets the hypothalamic temperature regulating center. NSAIDs suppress the formation of PGE2.
* *Analgesic action*: Prostaglandins sensitize the nerve endings to inflammatory mediators like bradykinin and 5 HT. NSAIDs prevent such sensitization by inhibiting prostaglandin synthesis. Headache is also relieved due to suppression of vasodilator prostaglandins.
* *Miscellaneous action*: For conversion of glucose to sorbitol, aldole reductase is required, which can be depressed by NSAIDs like sulindac and so it is being tried in the management of diabetic cataract and peripheral neuropathy. Aspirin inhibits platelet aggregation.

Indications for Topical Application

- Used before intraocular surgery for maintenance of blood aqueous barrier and mydriasis.
- Post-operative inflammation – used both as a preventive measure and also as a curative measure- either alone or synergistically with low dose topical steroid.
- Both therapeutic and refractive laser photokeratectomy – used as analgesic.
- Radial keratotomy – used as analgesic.
- Used in both the prevention and therapy of post operative cystoid macular edema.
- Used after removal of corneal foreign bodies.
- NSAIDs are used in various other conditions like anterior uveitis, episcleritis, scleritis, chemical injury to eye, acute inflammation produced by secondary glaucoma, vascularisation of cornea, etc.
- Ketorolac (0.5%) has been found to be very effective in the management of allergic conjunctivitis.

Indications for Systemic Application

- Systemic NSAIDs are successfully used in following ocular conditions:
  (i)   Uveitis.
  (ii) CME (but topical therapy is possibly more effective).
  (iii) Vernal keratoconjunctivitis.
  (iv) Scleritis and episcleritis.
- Aspirin by virtue of its property of inhibiting platelet aggregation has been tried successfully in:
  (i)   Retinal vascular occlusive diseases.
  (ii) Amaurosis fugax.
- Low dose aspirin might prevent development of cataract.

Side Effects

Topical application

- Local burning sensation and irritation
- Delay in regeneration of corneal epithelium

- Swelling of lids
- Conjunctival congestion
- Flurbiprofen type of NSAID may antagonize the IOP lowering effect of epinephrine but it has no effect on IOP lowering property of timolol and apraclonidine.

Systemic application

- Starting from gastric mucosal ulceration up to perforation. This side effect is due to inhibition of COX –1 which leads to suppression of production of gastric mucosa protective prostaglandin.
- Alopecia.
- Bone marrow depression.
- Hepatic and renal dysfunction.
- Edema associated with cardiac dysfunction.
- Blurring of vision, tinitus and hearing impairment.
- Occasionally, allergic reactions (most dangerous Stevens-Johnson syndrome), vertigo and headache, lethargy, etc.
- According to modern concept of human bronchial asthma, role of leukotrienes (LTs) is very crucial. Now if the COX pathway is blocked, the LOX pathway with its end products becomes hyperactive and there is precipitation of acute bronchial asthma in susceptible subjects.

Absolute Contraindications of NSAIDs

- Peptic ulcer
- Haematological disorder
- Hypersensitivity

Some Important NSAIDs

Diflunisal

It is a long acting salicylate containing fluorine. Although it is three times more potent than aspirin, it possesses no antipyretic property. The gastric irritation property is less and there occurs no tinitus. Further, it possesses uricosuric property.

Ketorolac

Although an NSAID, it has been successfully used in the management of allergic conjunctivitis (0.5% eye drop) to reduce ocular pruritus. Its analgesic property is comparable with that of morphine but no addiction property is noted.

Naproxen

It is a propionic acid derivative (Fig. 10.2) and is a potent NSAID which inhibits leukocyte migration and is the drug of choice in acute gout and ankylosing spondylitis.

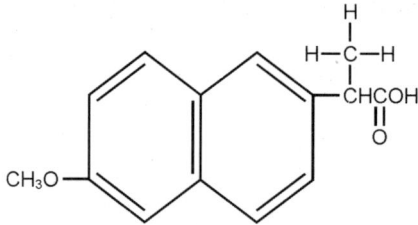

Fig. 10.2. Chemical structure of naproxen

Sulindac

It is a prodrug, chemically similar to indomethacin. In the body, it is converted into sulindac sulfide which is the active form of the compound. It is a selective inhibitor of extra-renal prostaglandin synthesis. It does not interfere with antihypertensive and diuretic action of beta blockers, ACE inhibitors and thiazides. It reduces the number and size of adenomas in those patients who have familial adenomatous polyposis.

Nabumetone

It is a prodrug and is converted in the body into its active metabolite which is a very potent COX-2 inhibitor. Its gastric irritation property is the minimum.

Mephenamic acid

It is mostly used as analgesic agent in soft tissue, muscle and joint pains. Its anti-inflammatory action is very poor.

Ibuprofen

It is a propionic acid derivative (Fig. 10.3) and is regarded as the safest conventional NSAID.

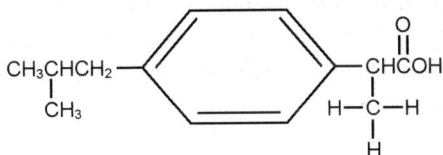

Fig. 10.3. Chemical structure of ibuprofen

Paracetamol

Paracetamol (Fig. 10.4) is a poor anti-inflammatory compound as it cannot inhibit prostaglandin synthesis in peripheral tissue, but is more powerful inhibitor of COX in brain and so acts as a good analgesic antipyretic compound.

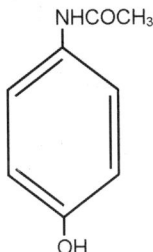

Fig. 10.4. Chemical structure of paracetamol

Rofecoxib

It is a selective COX-2 inhibitor. It is a powerful anti-inflammatory agent with practically no gastric irritation. It is contraindicated in hepato-renal diseases and hypertension. It has incompatibility with rifampicin, warfarin, methotrexate, etc.

Nimesulide

It is a powerful NSAID, effective in short lasting pathological conditions. A few cases of acute hepatic failure have recently been reported.

Oxicams

Oxicams are anti-inflammatory drugs with minimum gastric irritation. They reduce production of IgM rheumatoid factor and suppress chemotaxis of leucocytes and also decrease the ratio of T-helper to T-suppressor lymphocytes. Thus, oxicams can be regarded as broad spectrum anti-inflammatory agents. In this group, meloxicam is a specific COX-2 inhibitor.

Aspirin

In low doses, aspirin (Fig. 10.5) inhibits TXA2 synthesis in platelets and as a result, platelet aggregation is prevented and bleeding time is prolonged. This phenomenon is utilized in ocular therapeutics in the management of retinal vascular occlusive diseases and amaurosis fugax.

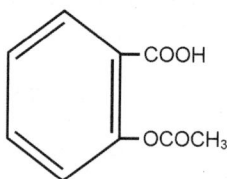

Fig. 10.5. Chemical structure of aspirin

Diclofenac

Diclofenac (Fig. 10.6) is an NSAID having analgesic, antipyretic and anti-inflammatory properties. Apart from inhibiting prostaglandin, it also suppresses neutrophil chemotaxis and development of superoxide. About 99% of the drug is protein bound. However, concurrent administration of lithium and digoxin may raise their blood levels.

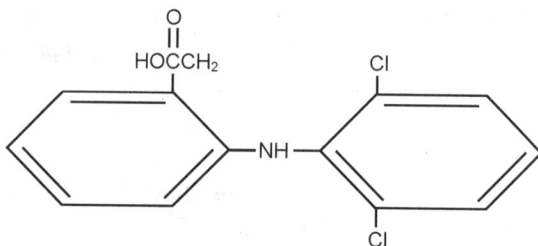

Fig. 10.6. Chemical structure of diclofenac

Nefopam

It is a benzoxazocine derivative, classified under non-opioid analgesics possessing no anti PG activity. It is a powerful analgesic (comparable with morphine), suitable for treating traumatic and post-operative musculoskeletal pain. It can produce anticholinergic, sympathomimetic side effects. It should not be used in epileptics.

Preparation and Dosage of Commonly Used NSAIDs

Topical preparations

Flurbiprofen 0.03%, suprofen 1%, diclofenac 0.1% and ketorolac tromethamine 0.5% are used as eye drops – 1 drop four times a day × 12 weeks or even more.

Systemic preparations

The doses are: Ibuprofen – 800 mg thrice daily, Diclofenac – 75 mg twice daily, Piroxicam – 20 mg four times a day, Sulindac – 150 mg twice daily, Indomethacin – 75 mg twice daily, Diflunisal – 500 mg twice daily or thrice daily, Naproxen – 250 mg to 500 mg twice daily, Aspirin – 500 mg to 1000 mg twice daily (but antithrombotic dose is only 50 to 100 mg per day), Tolmetin – 400 mg thrice daily.

Some Important Drug Interaction Related to NSAIDs

- Bleeding time is prolonged, when administered with anticoagulants.
- Antihypertensive action of beta blockers may be reduced.
- Serum level of lithium may be increased.
- Serum hydantoin levels may be increased leading to toxic manifestations.
- Naproxen and indomethacin may reduce antihypertensive and diuretic action of thiazide diuretics.
- Ibuprofen and indomethacin may increase serum level of digoxin.
- Indomethacin when administered with sympathomimetic drugs may increase blood pressure. It can also inhibit the effect of ACE inhibiters and can induce renal failure when used along with triamterene.

- Rofecoxib is incompatible with rifampicin, methotrexate and warfarin.

Some Special Toxicities Related to NSAIDs

Salicylism

Long continuous intake of salicylates may produce a condition called salicylism where the plasma level is found to be more than 25 mg per cent. The important characteristic features are headache, vertigo, tinitus, G.I. tract irritation, and visual and auditory impairment. There may be tachypnoea and respiratory alkalosis also. However, all these features are reversible on cessation of therapy.

Reye's syndrome

In children below 12 years, suffering from viral infection (e.g. influenza), administration of aspirin is contraindicated as it may precipitate hepatic encephalopathy, which is usually fatal.

Paracetamol poisoning

A large dose of paracetamol may produce necrosis of liver cells and renal tubular cells (condition is usually fatal). The condition develops due to accumulation of a metabolite of paracetamol called N-acetyl-p-benzoquinoneimine (NABQI), which causes depletion of hepatic glutathione and the metabolite binds to liver cells and renal tubular cells producing their necrosis.

N-acetylcysteine is the specific antidote for such a condition; it replenishes the hepatic glutathione stores and prevents the covalent binding of the toxic metabolites to liver cells and renal tubules. But N-acetylcysteine cannot counteract NABQI, if the treatment is started 16 hours after the ingestion of paracetamol.

Nimesulide

Many cases of fulminant hepatic failure have recently been reported recently and it has been withdrawn in many countries like Finland, Turkey, Spain, etc.

Piroxicam

Many cases of reversible azotemia have been reported with the use of piroxicam.

Synergistic action of NSAID and corticosteroids

They produce synergistic action. Moreover, the conditions where corticosteroid is absolutely necessary, the dose required is smaller (when used with NSAIDs).

Guidelines for Management of Some Important Ocular Conditions where Topical NSAIDs Are Used

- Flurbiprofen (0.03%) eye drop is particularly useful in preventing intra-operative miosis. It has a good corneal penetration power and for best results it should be used 4-6 times just before surgery.
- Diclofenac (0.1%) eye drop is a very good drug for preventing cystoid macular edema.
- Ketorolac (0.5%) eye drop has been successfully used to manage itching of all allergic conjunctivitis.
- Indomethacin (0.5% to 1%) eye drop is a brilliant drug for prevention of intra-operative miosis. For best results, 1 drop 4 times (at 15 minutes intervals) one hour prior to extra-capsular cataract surgery is used. It is also used at 6 hourly intervals after the surgery for prevention of post-operative inflammation.

CHAPTER 11

Parasympathomimetics

Certain drugs act through stimulation or mimicking of the parasympathetic nervous system (PNS). Hence, these are called parasympathomimetics. These are also called cholinergics because acetylcholine (ACh) is the neurotransmitter used by the PNS. The effects of parasympathomimetic drugs resemble the effects produced by stimulation of parasympathetic (cholinergic) nervous system.

The parasympathomimetic drugs can act in two ways:

(i) Directly by stimulating the nicotinic or muscarinic receptors, or

(ii) Indirectly by inhibiting cholinesterase, promoting acetylcholine release, or through other mechanisms.

The cholinergic receptors are classified into two broad groups:

1. *Muscarinic receptors*: Five subtypes M_1, M_2, M_3, M_4 and M_5 have been recognized, out of which M_1, M_2 and M_3 are more well-defined. M_1 is present in CNS, gastric glands, autonomic ganglia, etc., M_2 in heart; and M_3 in visceral smooth muscles, exocrine glands, vascular endothelium, etc.

2. *Nicotinic receptors*: Two subtypes have been recognized, N_M is found in neuromuscular junction and N_N in autonomic ganglia, adrenal medulla, CNS, etc.

Stimulation of muscarinic receptors in eye results in miosis (constriction of pupil), spasm of accommodation (due to contraction of ciliary muscles) and fall of IOP (particularly in glaucoma subjects).

Classification of Parasympathomimetic Drugs Used In Ophthalmology Practice

I.Directly acting parasympathomimetics (Muscarinic receptor agonists):
- (a) Choline esters, e.g., Acetylcholine, Carbachol, Methacholine, etc.
- (b) Cholinomimetic alkaloids, e.g., Pilocarpine.
- (c) Some miscellaneous compounds, e.g., Aceclidine, Oxotremorine, etc.

II. Indirectly acting parasympathomimetics (Anticholinesterases):
- (a) Reversible anticholinesterases, e.g., Physostigmine, Neostigmine, Edrophonium, Demecarium, etc.
- (b) Irreversible anticholinesterases, e.g., Echothiophate, Diisopropyl – fluoro-phosphate (DFP).

Some Important Parasympathomimetics

Directly Acting Parasympathomimetics

Acetylcholine

Acetylcholine (Fig. 11.1) has very short half life and, hence, is not used as an antiglaucoma agent. But it is used as an intra-operative miotic agent.

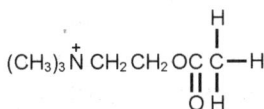

$$(CH_3)_3 \overset{+}{N} CH_2 CH_2 OC \overset{\overset{H}{|}}{\underset{\underset{O}{||} \underset{H}{|}}{C}} - H$$

Fig. 11.1. Chemical structure of acetylcholine

Carbachol

Carbachol (Fig. 11.2) is more stable than acetycholine and is not easily destroyed by cholinesterase, but it causes insignificant inhibition

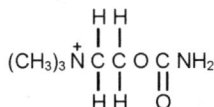

$$(CH_3)_3 \overset{+}{N} \overset{\overset{H}{|}}{\underset{\underset{H}{|}}{C}} \overset{\overset{H}{|}}{\underset{\underset{H}{|}}{C}} O \overset{}{\underset{\underset{O}{||}}{C}} NH_2$$

Fig. 11.2. Chemical structure of carbachol

of cholinesterase. It is lipid-insoluble. So, its penetration requires wetting agents like benzalkonium chloride or viscous carrier substance (like methyl cellulose). It is used as an anti-glaucoma agent (0.75%, 1.5%, 2.25%, 3% solutions are available) and is more powerful than pilocarpine both as a miotic and an IOP lowering agent. Moreover, its duration of action is also long. Usual dose is 1 drop twice or thrice daily. Intracamerally (0.01%), it acts as a powerful miotic.

Pilocarpine

Previously, pilocarpine (Fig. 11.3) was the most popular anti-glaucoma drug. It is an alkaloid derived from Pilocarpus microphyllus. Appreciable amount is absorbed after topical application.

   Its anti-glaucoma action takes place by facilitating aqueous outflow by stimulating longitudinal muscle fibres of ciliary body and thus by its contraction a tractional force is exerted on scleral spur. In closed angle glaucoma, miosis helps to improve the facility of aqueous outflow by relieving pupillary block. [N.B. Sometimes, due to contraction of ciliary muscles, the lens zonule gets relaxed and there is forward displacement of iris lens diaphragm which may cause an acute attack of closed angle glaucoma].

   Onset of action of 2% pilocarpine eye drop (ocular hypotensive action) starts within 20 to 45 minutes and lasts up to 6-8 hours. Higher concentration is needed in dark pigmented eyes. It increases thickness of lens (axial length) and thus causes myopia (pilocarpine induced). Intra-ocular tension drops 8-9 mm Hg with 2% solution. Higher concentration does not affect magnitude of fall of IOP but affects duration (up to 12 hours approximately).

Dosage: Pilocarpine nitrate is available as 1%, 2% & 4% solutions. Different types of preparations are available, like drops, ocusert

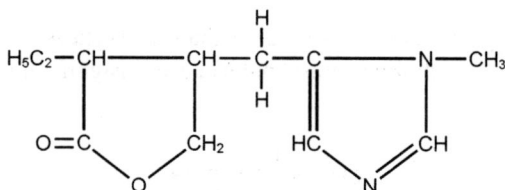

Fig. 11.3. Chemical structure of pilocarpine

(controlled release system) and gel form (4%). The usual dosage is 1 drop, 2 to 4 times a day.
Side effects: Side effects of pilocarpine are summarized in Table 11.1.

Table 11.1. Side effects of pilocarpine

Systemic effects	Ocular effects
1. Usually mild salivation, sweating, nausea, vomiting, diarrhoea, lacrimation, etc.	1. Decreased vision in low illumination due to stimulation of iris sphincter.
2. Serious effects are bronchiolar spasm and pulmonary edema.	2. Misleading field defect due to decline in threshold sensitivity.
[N.B. Multiple instillation of drops during acute attack of angle closure glaucoma produces no miosis (due to Sphinter pupillae paralysis) and increases risk of systemic toxicity].	3. Severe supra-orbital and temporal headache due to ciliary spasm.
	4. Induced myopia.
	5. Myotic cyst formation (simultaneous application of phenyl ephrine 2.5% solution may prevent this complication).
	6. Drug allergy.
	7. Retinal detachment
	8. It may have some cataractogenic effect.

Aceclidine

It is a synthetic cholinergic drug resembling pilocarpine in action; it produces very less amount of ciliary spasm (hence less induced axial myopia). It is very much suitable for young people. A 2% solution, 1 drop BID or QID is used.

Oxotremorine

It is a newer drug – M2 receptor agonist -- which improves outflow facilities without appreciable effect on pupil and accommodation. It is still under trial and not available for therapeutic use.

Indirectly Acting Parasympathomimetics

Reversible anticholinesterases

Cholinesterase is a non-specific type of enzyme which is present at all cholinergic sites, red blood cells, grey matter, etc. It acts on acetylcholine to divide it into acetyl CoA and choline and thus terminates its action.

Anticholinesterases are the drugs which competitively inhibit action of cholinesterase and cause sustained action of acetylcholine on its receptor site. So in short, it prolongs the action of acetylcholine.

Physostigmine

Physostigmine salicylate (Fig. 11.4) is the salicylate of an alkaloid obtained from the seeds of Physostigma venenosum.

Dosage: Physostigmine salicylate 0.25%-0.5%, 1 drop twice or thrice daily; Physostigmin sulphate solution 0.25%, 1 drop twice or thrice daily.

Therapeutic uses:

- Used as miotic and antiglaucoma agent.
- In anticholinergic drug poisoning. The usual dose is 0.5 mg to 1 mg orally not exceeding a dose of 3 mg, or alternatively 0.5 mg I.M. may be used.

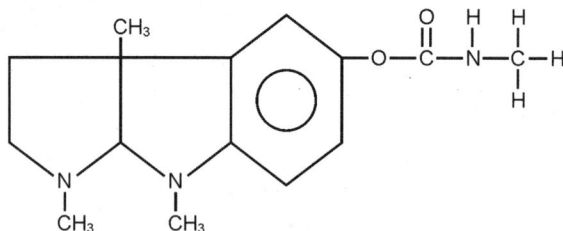

Fig.11.4. Chemical structure of physostigmine

Neostigmine

Neostigmine is a synthetic compound (Fig. 11.5). The dose is Neostigmine methyl sulphate solution 0.25% - 1%, 1 drop three or four times daily.

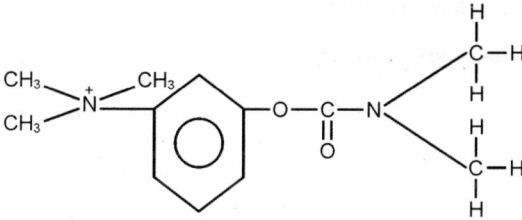

Fig. 11.5. Chemical structure of neostigmine

Its therapeutic use is similar to that of physostigmine, but neostigmine is more effective for the diagnosis of myasthenia gravis. Subcutaneous injection 0.5 mg of neostigmine promptly (usually within 15 minutes) improves diplopia, ptosis, general muscular weakness and other features of myasthenia gravis.

Toxicity: Physostigmine and neostigmine share the same signs and symptoms of toxicities, such as lacrimation, vomiting, diarrhea, abdominal cramp, bradycardia, etc. But the most dangerous features are respiratory depression, pulmonary edema and violent convulsions.

Edrophonium

Edrophonium (Fig. 11.6) has both anticholinesterase and direct neuromuscular stimulating effects. Its only ophthalmic use is diagnosis of myasthenia gravis. Other important use is in post-operative decurarisation.

Dosage: Edrophonium chloride, 1-10 mg I.V.

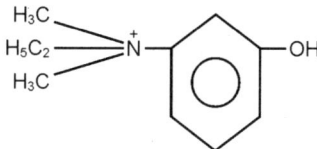

Fig. 11.6. Chemical structure of edrophonium

Demecarium bromide

It is a condensation product of two neostigmine molecules linked by a chain of 10 methylene groups. It is a potent long acting miotic, available as 0.125%-0.25% eye drop. Miosis lasts for about 1-3 days.

Irreversible anticholinesterases

Echothiophate (Phospholine)

Echothiophate (Phospholine) (Fig. 11.7) is an irreversible anti-cholinesterase compound. Solutions lose potency very quickly, so it is dispensed in powder form (only freshly prepared solutions are used). Facility of outflow is increased (about 135%); peak action is after about 24 hours, which may persist up to approximately 4 days. A solution containing 0.03% is potent and at the same time least toxic. The range of dose is 0.03%-0.25%, 1 drop/ day or on alternate days. *Systemic toxicities*: Nausea, abdominal cramps, general fatigue, diarrhea, etc. These can be treated by specific antidotes–cholinesterase reactivators (oximes).

Ocular toxicities: Corneal endothelial changes (reversible and dose dependent), iris cyst (preventable, if used with phenylephrine), iritis, cataract (dose-dependant), retinal detachment, etc.

Therapeutic uses:

• Open angle glaucoma
• Accommodative esotropia

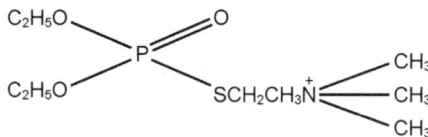

Fig. 11.7. Chemical structure of echothiophate

Di-isopropyl fluorophosphate (DFP)

Di-isopropyl fluorophosphate (DFP) (Fig. 11.8) is dispensed as 0.01%-0.1% oily solution since water rapidly inactivates it.

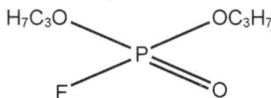

Fig. 11.8. Chemical structure of DFP

CHAPTER 12

Antimuscarinic Drugs

These drugs block the muscarinic receptor mediated response of parasympathetic nervous system. They can be classified as:

I. Natural alkaloids, e.g., Atropine (obtained from Atropa belladonna and Datura stramonium) and Hyoscine (Scopolamine) obtained from Hyoscyamus niger.

II. Synthetic compounds, e.g., Homatropine, Cyclopentolate and Tropicamide

Natural Alkaloids

Atropine

Atropine (Fig. 12.1) has many pharmacological actions in whole body. Here only ophthalmological actions will be discussed in details. Its main actions on eye are mydriasis and cycloplegia. When applied, it takes 30-40 min for mydriasis to occur which lasts at least for 12 days. Similarly, cycloplegia takes a few hours to occur and lasts for 2 weeks or even longer. (N.B. Usually, phenylephrine types of

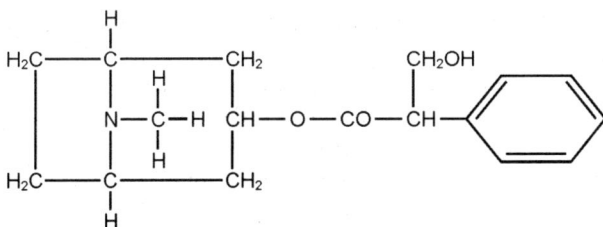

Fig. 12.1. Chemical structure of atropine

sympathomimetics are prescribed along with atropine. In mydriasis they act synergistically but for cycloplegia, the sympathomimetic has insignificant action).

Other actions

Tear flow: The flow is definitely reduced but there is no change in formation of lysozyme and tear protein. Hence tear gets more concentrated.

Pigmentation: Atropine melanin binding theory has been postulated as pupil dilate very slowly and cycloplegia also takes some time, but durations of both are prolonged in deeply pigmented eyes.

Therapeutic uses

(A) *In Iridocyclitis*: Atropine is the drug of choice in acute iridocyclitis.
    (a) It leads to reduction of pain by giving complete relaxation to inflamed musculature of iris and ciliary body.
    (b) Posterior synechiae is the most sight threatening complication in acute iridocyclitis. Atropine (1% solution applied thrice daily) along with Phynylephrine (10% eye drop) gives adequate relief. Sometimes, sub-conjunctival injection of mydricaine (a mixture of atropine, procaine and adrenaline) is helpful.
    (c) Atropine stabilizes the blood eye barrier and thereby reduces abnormal types of vascular permeabilities.

(B) *For refraction purposes:*Atropine refraction is necessary in children, particularly in squint cases.

(C) *In Hyphaema:* It has been observed that there is no difference in visual outcome, rate of absorption of blood or secondary haemorrhage, whether atropine has been used or not. However, ophthalmologists get better view of inner eye and patients usually feel comfortable if atropine is used.

(D) *As a premedication agent:* Atropine injection 0.4 mg I.M., as a premedication agent, usually prevents oculocardiac reflex which occurs due to vagal stimulation during strabismus surgery. There may be slowing of heart rate, hypertension, nausea and even fainting attack. It may also occur in ptosis or in entropion surgery.

Side effects

Side effects are dry mouth, difficulty in talking, fever, allergic rash, blurring of vision, excitement, cardiovascular collapse, convulsion, etc.

Among the ocular side effects, it may precipitate acute glaucoma in anatomically narrow angle individuals. Atropine hypertensitivity may occur in some individuals that can be treated effectively by corticosteroid ointment.

Toxicity

Lethal dose in children is 10-20 mg (in adults 80-130 mg). So, a single vial of 1% atropine drops can kill many children. It should be kept safely beyond the reach of children.

In case of accidental poisoning:

- Gastric lavage should be given with activated charcoal.
- Patient should be placed in a dark comfortable room.
- Ice bags, cold sponging and antifebrile agents should be used.
- Its specific antidote is physostigmine 1-3 mg given subcutaneously or intravenously (depending on severity), which effectively counteracts both central and peripheral action. The dose may have to be repeated after 4-6 hours. Neostigmine has been found to be less effective than physostigmine. In children, the dose of physostigmine used is 0.5-1 mg.
- Supportive measures like fluid transfusion, artificial respiration, diazepam (10 mg), I.V. inj. (to control convulsions if any), etc., should be started immediately.

Scopolamine

It is a natural alkaloid (Fig. 12.2) obtained from Hyoscyamus niger. It is available in 0.1% to 0.5% solution. Time taken for full mydriasis to occur is after 20 minutes of instillation. It then starts decreasing rapidly and the effect totally passes off after 8 days. Time taken for cycloplegia to occur after instillation is about 40 min (after instillation). The cycloplegic effect passes off very quickly. Side effects are more or less similar to those of atropine but psychotic effect is more common in this case. In contrast to atropine, scopolamine is CNS-depressant.

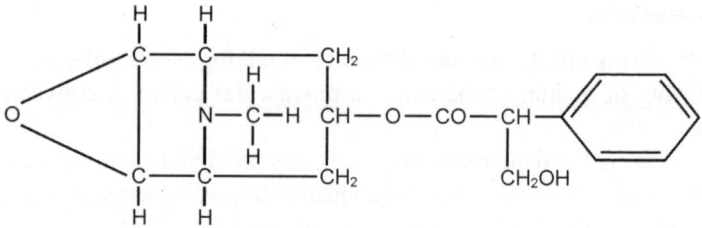

Fig. 12.2. Chemical structure of scopolamine

Synthetic Compounds

Homatropine

It is 10 times less potent than atropine; 1% and 2% eye drops are more commonly used. Time taken for full mydriasis and cycloplegia to occur is 45-60 min and the effect lasts for 1-3 days. It is used in adults. In children, it causes incomplete cycloplegia. When used in normal therapeutic dose, practically no side effect is seen. It is usually used for refraction purpose in adults.

Cyclopentolate

This synthetic compound is a very potent mydriatic and cycloplegic drug. Usually, 0.5% - 1% solution is used. Both mydriasis and cycloplegia in full form are seen within 30-60 min and usually last for a day or two.

It is best avoided in patient with history of uveitis as it has a chemotactic effect on leucocytes. As is seen with other mydriatics, cyclopentolate may cause rise in I.O.P., in both open and closed angle glaucoma cases. It is avoided in children as it may produce a peculiar type of psychotic reaction in them. Sometimes, it may produce topical allergic reactions. It is used for refraction purposes, and in milder cases of anterior uveitis.

Tropicamide

It is available as 0.5%-1% solution. It is most rapidly acting mydriatic (20-40 min) (cycloplegic action unpredictable) and the duration of action is also very short (3-6 hours). Side effects are rare. However, it may also cause (like other mydriatics) transient rise of I.O.P. in closed angle glaucoma subjects. Very rarely, it may produce psychotic reactions and circulatory collapse. It is mainly used for the purpose of refraction in adults and indirect ophthalmoscopy (along with phenylephrine).

CHAPTER 13

Sympathomimetic Drugs

Sympathomimetic drugs are those drugs whose effects resemble the effect of stimulation of sympathetic nervous system depending on the type of receptor concerned.

Adrenergic receptors are of two types: alpha and beta. Alpha receptors have been subdivided on pharmacological basis into alpha 1 and alpha 2. Recently, during molecular cloning, further subdivisions have been suggested; in the case of alpha 1 receptors: alpha 1A, alpha 1B and alpha 1D, and in the case of alpha 2 receptors: alpha 2A, alpha 2B and alpha 2C.

Beta receptors are of 3 types – beta 1 (present in heart and kidney), beta 2 (present in eye, bronchi, blood vessels, uterus, G.I. tract and urinary tract) and beta 3 receptors (present in adipose tissue)

Common Sympathomimetic Drugs

The common sympathomimetic drugs used in ophthalmology are:
- Epinephrine
- Dipivalyl epinephrine
- Phenylephrine
- Hydroxy amphetamine
- Clonidine
- Apraclonidine
- Brimonidine
- Ibopamine

Epinephrine

Epinephrine (Fig. 13.1) increases outflow of aqueous humour. The possible mechanisms involved are:

(a) Beta 2 receptor stimulation leads to 20% increase in uveoscleral outflow.

(b) Later, there is alpha 2 receptor stimulation, which leads to increased uveoscleral or trabecular outflow.

(c) It influences cell shape and cell-to-cell contact, increasing trabecular outflow.

(d) Epinephrine interferes with bio-synthesis of glycosaminoglycan in the trabecular meshwork and causes depolymerization of action filaments in trabecular meshwork. These factors further improve the outflow.

(e) Indirectly, it stimulates endogenous prostaglandin synthesis and thereby increases uveoscleral outflow.

Dosage

1% to 2% solution is used, twice daily initially, followed by once daily in the morning as maintenance dose (as IOP remains low even for a few weeks after the initial loading dose).

Action starts within 1 hour of instillation, maximum peak action after 4 hours of instillation, action lasts up to 12-24 hours after the last application. Epinephrine may fail to reduce IOP in 30% glaucoma cases, the cause of which is unknown.

Use as mydriatic: If a cotton pack is placed in the lower conjunctival fornix pre-soaked with epinephrine, (1 in 1000) full dilatation of pupil occurs. It is particularly useful for breaking posterior synechiae. It is also used with miotics to make pupil slightly larger to provide a little better vision.

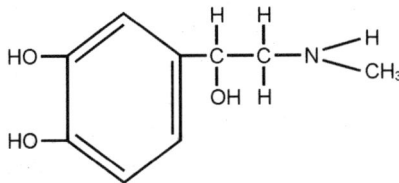

Fig. 13.1. Chemical structure of epinephrine

Use as local vasoconstrictor:

(a) Epinephrine constricts capillaries and small arterioles, but is ineffective in bleeding from larger vessels. So, to avoid irritating capillary oozing during surgery, epinephrine is used as a topical solution (1 in 1000) just prior to operation. Its action as vasoconstrictor starts within 5 minutes and the effect lasts for about an hour.

(b) In the concentration of 1 in 200,000, it can be mixed with local anaesthetic preparation for injection purposes. It will lead to less bleeding at the site of incision. Moreover, it retards the rate of absorption of local anaesthetics at the operative site.

(c) A drop of topical epinephrine causing quick disappearance of congestion of a red eye indicates superficial congestion.

Ocular side effects

A slight burning sensation, congestion and eye ache are common side effects. More serious side effects include corneal edema, drug allergy, pigmentary changes in the conjunctiva, maculopathy, retinal haemorrhage, cystoid macular degeneration, reactivation of herpes keratitis and iatrogenic pemphigoid.

Prolonged use (for more than one year) causes deposition of an oxidative breakdown product of epinephrine, called adrenochrome pigment (dark brown or black) within translucent conjunctival cyst. It is commonly seen in old people.

Epinephrine maculopathy is usually seen in aphakic eyes treated with epinephrine (about 20% to 30% aphakics are affected). Features may start within a few weeks to a few months of starting the medication. If diagnosed at a little late stage, it is often associated with cystoid degeneration and haemorrhage around macula. Discontinuation of therapy usually leads to return of vision, which may take even 6 months. But if associated with features of degeneration (diagnosed lately), some visual acuity is lost permanently. Biomicroscopy and fluorescein angiography are enough to confirm the diagnosis. It has been curiously observed that in cases with intact posterior capsule, the incidence is much less (as less epinephrine reaches choroid). The possible reasons for such maculopathy formation may be as follows:

*   Increased prostaglandin synthesis by epinephrine.
*   About 80% reduction in protein synthesis due to combined action of epinephrine and ultraviolet rays of sun.
*   Diminished blood flow in uveal tissue (due to alpha effect of epinephrine).

Systemic side effects

Milder side effects are extrasystoles, tachycardia, palpitation, etc. The patients with coronary heart disease, thyrotoxicosis, hypertension, diabetes, etc., are more prone to get these toxicities.

General anaesthetics like cyclopropane or halothane sensitize the myocardium more to epinephrine and so cardiac arrhythmias are very common if these drugs are used in a patient on topical epinephrine therapy.

Dipivefrin

It is a prodrug (inactive biologically) which gets converted into an active drug molecule (epinephrine) with the help of tissue enzymes present in cornea. It is more lipid-soluble than epinephrine and so its corneal penetration power is 17 times more than that of epinephrine. After instillation, the ocular hypotensive action starts within 30 minutes and reaches its peak at the end of 1 hour.

A 0.1% solution is used once in the morning. However, it may be used twice daily also.

Its side effects include allergy (local) and maculopathy. Conjunctival pigmentation does not occur and systemic toxicities are rare.

Phenylephrine

Phenylephrine (Fig. 13.2) is a selective alpha 1 receptor agonist. It causes mydriasis, vasoconstriction and fall in I.O.P. (But in anatomically narrow angle, it may produce an acute attack of glaucoma).

Dosage

It is available as 2.5-10% solution. With a single instillation of 2.5%-5% solution, maximum dilatation occurs within 60-90 minutes and

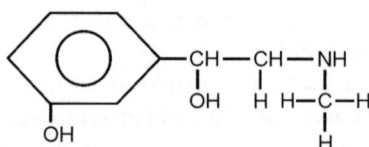

Fig.13.2. Chemical structure of phenylephrine

stays for 5-7 hours. But 10% solution causes a little more dilatation and the duration of action increases.

Prodrug

Phenylephrine oxazolin is a prodrug, which can be used in the place of phenylephrine. It possesses more corneal penetration capacity and has more therapeutic efficacy in low dose.

Antagonist of phenylephrine

Alpha 1 antagonist like dapiprazole or thymoxamine can block its action.

Therapeutic uses of phenylephrine

- Used as a mydriatic (even 2.5% solution is capable).
- Used along with miotics to prevent miotic cyst formation.
- Used as conjunctival vasoconstrictor (0.125% solution).

Contraindications

- Infants (severe hypertension with subarachnoid haemorrhage has been reported).
- Narrow angle glaucoma.
- Coronary heart disease.
- Hyperthyroidism.
- Diabetic individuals with autonomic nervous system dysfunction.
- Hypertensive individuals.

Hydroxyamphetamine

It is an indirectly acting sympathomimetic agent, used as a 1% topical solution. It depletes norepinephrine from adrenergic nerve terminals.

Its effect can be counteracted by guanethidine (adrenergic neuron blocking agent). In normal eyes it causes rapid mydriasis. In central and preganglionic lesion induced Horner's syndrome, it produces pupillary dilatation (as endogenous epinephrine is present), whereas in postganglionic lesion induced Horner's syndrome, pupillary dilatation does not occur.

Clonidine

Clonidine (Fig. 13.3) is an antiglaucoma drug, having practically no effect on accommodation and pupillary diameter. The concentration used is 0.0625%, 0.125% or 0.25%, 1 drop twice or thrice daily; duration of action of single application lasts for about 6 to 8 hours.

Mechanism of antiglaucoma action

(a) It stimulates alpha 2 receptors, which leads to suppression of norepinephrine release. As a result, there is reduction of stimulation of beta receptors and consequently there is reduction in the formation of cyclic AMP and suppression of aqueous formation.

(b) There is improvement in uveoscleral or trabecular outflow and reduction in episcleral venous pressure.

(c) There is associated local vasoconstriction, probably by non-specific alpha 1 effect.

It has been observed that there is a fall in IOP of both eyes even if the drug is applied to one eye possibly due to a little amount of accumulation of the drug in the other eye also.

Adverse reactions

• Fall of blood pressure, particularly in hypertensives.

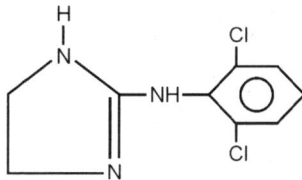

Fig. 13.3. Chemical structure of clonidine

- As there is decrease in local perfusion pressure of the eye, so there is a chance of slight impairment of perfusion of optic nerve head. However, it has been experimentally observed (pulsatile blood flow studies) that there is an increase in the total blood flow, which is beyond expectation and does not tally with the amount of fall in IOP.
- A slight conjunctival irritation, blanching and hyperaemia, etc., are observed.
- Initially, there may be a slight dryness of mouth and sedation.

Apraclonidine

Apraclonidine (Fig. 13.4) is a less-selective alpha 2 stimulator. It has practically no effect on systemic B.P. It has a drawback that on prolonged use, it may give rise to allergic manifestation (local) in 50% cases and so the medication has to be given up in the mid way. Therefore, it is mainly used as a short term medication, e.g., management of IOP after anterior segment laser surgery, prior to cataract extraction as an adjuvant with mydriatics (with anatomical narrow angle), etc. Mechanism of anti-glaucoma action is similar to that in the case of clonidine. Systemic side effects are similar to those of clonidine (except that it has no effect on BP) and local side effects are also similar to those of clonidine (in addition to ocular allergy as already discussed).

Its concentration used in therapeutics varies from 0.25% to 1%. In prophylactic use, 1 drop is administered before laser treatment and another drop after the procedure is over. If desired for long term therapy, 1 drop of 0.25% to 0.5% solution is instilled bid or tid. For short term therapy, 1 drop of 1% solution tid or bid may be used.

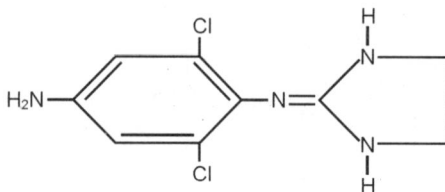

Fig. 13.4. Chemical structure of apraclonidine

Brimonidine

It is a specific alpha 2 agonist. The mechanism of action of IOP lowering effect is similar to that in the case of apraclonidine. In addition, it increases uveoscleral outflow. It has a neuroprotective function also.

Therapeutic use

- Management of acute IOP rise after argon laser trabeculoplasty.
- Management of glaucoma.
- For long term use, 0.2% solution –1 drop bid or tid.
- For prophylactic use, 0.5% solution –1 drop prior to procedure.

Side effects

- Systemic side effects include only dry mouth, sedation and fatigue sensation, but no cardiovascular or pulmonary effect. However, tachyphylaxis may be a problem in 20% of the patients.
- Local reactions include eye lid retraction, conjunctival blanching, and local allergic reaction.
- Contraindicated in the patients undergoing MAO inhibitor therapy.

Ibopamine

Pharmacologically it is a dopamine receptor stimulating drug. Its important uses in ophthalmic practice are:

- As an efficient mydriatic agent – 1% solution is used (It is best is to use it along with cyclopentolate to get a brilliant mydriasis).
- 1% solution is used as a provocative test for glaucoma (as it increases the aqueous production).
- In post-operative hypotonia, 2% solution is used.

CHAPTER 14

Adrenergic Antagonists

Adrenergic antagonists are chemicals that have high affinity for adrenergic receptors. They inhibit the effects of catecholamines by competing for andrenergic receptor sites and preventing endogenous catecholamines from exerting their effects. These antagonists inhibit specifically alpha, beta or dopaminergic adrenergic receptors.

Amongst the adrenergic antagonists, three groups of drugs are used with advantage in ophthalmology:

I. Alpha-1 antagonists, e.g., thymoxamine, dapiprazole, etc.
II. Beta blockers, e.g., timolol, betaxolol, levobunolol, metipranolol, carteolol, adaprolol, etc.
III. Miscellaneous antiadrenergic agents, e.g., guanethidine, 6-hydroxydopamine, etc.

Alpha-1 Antagonists

Thymoxamine and dapiprazole are topical alpha-1 blockers.

Thymoxamine

It is used in 0.1% and 0.5% solutions to produce miosis. It has got no action on IOP and accommodation.

Therapeutic use

*   For rapid counteraction of phenylephrine mydriasis. One can, therefore, examine the fundus of a narrow angle case without much risk. 0.5% solution is usually used.

- Hyperthyroid lid retracton. The condition improves within 15 minutes and duration of effect is approximately for a few hours when 0.5% solution is used.
- Prevention of the acute attack of narrow angle glaucoma. It has been found to prevent an impending acute attack of narrow angle glaucoma through frequent instillations (0.5%, 1 drop at 15 min intervals for a period of at least 2 to 3 hours).
- Pigmentary glaucoma. It has been found to be effective in pigmentary glaucoma.

Side effects

There may be a little conjunctival hyperaemia due to loss of vascular tone and a little ptosis.

Dapiprazole

Usually, a 0.5% solution is used.

Therapeutic use

- Reversal of mydriasis produced by phenylephrine, tropicamide, etc. Reversal is complete within 30 min. To some extent, it counteracts the cycloplegic action of tropicamide also.
- As it has been found to enhance the pressure lowering effect of timolol, it is used as an adjuvant with timolol.

Side effects

Conjunctival hyperaemia, corneal irritation, corneal edema (rarely), slower miotic action in darkly pigmented iris.

Beta-blockers of Ophthalmic Importance

Mechanism of Action of Beta-blockers in Eye

Mechanism of ocular hypotensive action of beta blockers is not yet very clear. However, possibilities are:

(a) There is inhibition in concentration of cyclic AMP in the ciliary epithelial cells due to blockage of beta 2 receptor resting tone and as a result of this, aqueous production is minimized (beta blockers have practically no effect on outflow which was believed in the past).

(b) Another possible mechanism of reduction of IOP is depression of Na^+, K^+, ATPase mechanism.

It is interesting to note that beta blockers act when the subject is awake by reducing the adrenergic stimulation (i.e. resting tone) and the IOP lowering is seen only when the subject is awake and conscious. Beta blockers, therefore, practically have no effect on IOP during sleep.

Timolol Maleate

It (Fig. 14.1) is a non-selective beta blocker. Topical preparations are 0.25% and 0.5% solutions to be instilled once or twice daily.

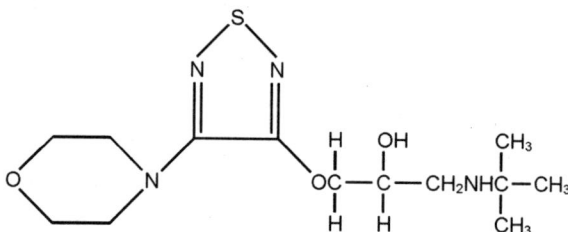

Fig. 14.1. Chemical structure of timolol

Betaxolol

It is a beta 1 specific antagonist. It is used as betaxolol hydrochloride, 0.25% and 0.5% solutions. As it is a selective beta 1 blocker, it is relatively safer (compared with timolol) to use in patients with ischaemia, bradycardia, depressed pulmonary function, etc. But still the present day concept is that beta blockers (whether beta 1 antagonist or beta 1 + beta 2 antagonist) should be avoided in patients having history of bronchospasm.

Levobunolol

It is used as a 0.25% or 0.5% solution (eye drop) once or twice daily.

Metipranolol

It is used as a 0.3% solution (eye drop) once or twice daily.

Carteolol

It is a hydrophilic non-selective beta blocker with intrinsic sympathomimetic activity. It is weaker than timolol and levobunolol. It is applied twice daily, 1% or 2% solution.

Adaprolol

It is one of the newer beta antagonists. A locally acting beta-blocker, it has a very short plasma half-life (about 7 min). It acts on local ocular tissues and is then quickly metabolized so that chances of systemic toxicity is practically nil. The suggested dose is 0.2% to 0.4%, twice daily. It is not yet available in open market.

Adverse Reactions of Beta-blockers

Local

- Dry eye syndrome (since the beta blockers destroy the tear film due to their membrane stabilizing and local anaesthetic properties).
- In addition, they inhibit the tear secretion, punctate keratopathy, and produce ocular and orbital pain.

Systemic

- Cardiovascular system – Slight bradycardia, hypotension, heart block, arrhythmia.
- Respiratory system – Acute bronchospasm, particularly in patients with past history of asthma.
- CNS – Mental depression, loss of memory, lack of libido, even hallucinations.
- Alimentary system – Nausea, vomiting, anorexia, diarrhoea, dry mouth, etc.
- Dermal system – Allergic rash, hyper pigmentation, alopecia, toxic epidermal necrolysis, etc.

- Endocrine system – Masking of features of hypoglycaemia in patients undergoing insulin therapy.
- General headache, fatigue, muscular asthenia, etc.

Contraindications

- Respiratory obstructive disease.
- Bronchial asthma.
- Heart block.

Important drug interactions

- Potentiation of the drug, if given to a patient who is already receiving oral beta blocker.
- Topical beta blocker if given to a patient who is on oral digitalis or calcium channel blocker therapy may cause prolongation of atrioventricular conduction time.
- Simultaneous administration of topical beta blocker and calcium channel blocker may precipitate hypotension and left ventricular failure (particularly in patients with deranged cardiac function).
- It may mask the features of acute hypoglycaemia (mediated through sympathetic stimulations like tremor, tachycardia) in patients receiving oral hypoglycaemic or insulin therapy.
- It may mask many features of thyrotoxicosis.
- Acute withdrawal of beta blockers in thyrotoxic patients may produce thyroid storm.

Miscellaneous Antiadrenergic Agents

Guanethidine

It is a sympatholytic drug which causes depletion of norepiephrine from sympathetic nerve terminals. A 10% topical solution has been used for cosmetic correction of lid retraction in thyrotoxic patients. The dose is 1 to 4 drops / day. One drop causes onset of action after 6 to 8 hours and the duration of action lasts for a few days. Systemically, it acts as an antihypertensive agent.

6-Hydroxydopamine

It is an isomer of norepinephrine. It causes selective degeneration of sympathetic nerve terminals without affecting any other nerve, the effect lasting for about 14 weeks. The process is called chemical sympathectomy. A sub-conjunctival injection is given (0.2 ml of 2% solution) at limbus (avoiding 12 o'clock position to avoid injury to Muller's muscle). The process is tried in absolute glaucoma cases.

CHAPTER 15

Antiglaucoma Drugs

Antiglaucoma drugs are covered under the following heads:
- Autonomic drugs (These have already been discussed in Chapters 11, 13 and 14).
- Prostaglandin derivatives.
- Carbonic anhydrase inhibitors.
- Hyperosmotic agents.
- Recent medications for glaucoma.
- Drugs used during glaucoma surgery.

Prostaglandin Derivatives

These generally work by increasing the uveoscleral outflow of aqueous humour.

Latanoprost

It is a prodrug which gets activated by esterase while passing through cornea. It has been recently approved by FDA. It should be used if conventional anti-glaucoma drugs fail or produce severe side effects.

Mechanism of action

Although the mechanism is not conclusively established, the general suggestions are as follows:
(a) There is increased facility of uveoscleral outflow, mediated via the stimulation of prostanoid receptor F.B. (situated in the ciliary muscle).

(b) A second hypothesis states that there is a slight increase in trabecular outflow.

Side effects

Side effects are few. They include conjunctival hyperaemia, increase in iris pigmentation and, very rarely superficial punctate keratopathy. The hyperpigmentation of iris is due to stimulation of iris stromal melanocytes, which produce more melanin.

Dosage

Suggested dosage is 0.005% solution – only 1 drop daily in the evening.

Unoprostone

It is another prostaglandin derivative less potent but less toxic than latanoprost. The only toxicity is superficial punctate keratopathy in isolated cases. The suggested concentration and dose is 0.12% - 1 drop twice daily.

Travoprost

It is one of latest drugs of this series. Available as 0.004% eye drop, it is used as 1 drop in the evening per day. It shares all the side effects of latanoprost. In addition, there is a chance of development of cystoid macular edema.

Carbon Anhydrase Inhibitors

These generally work by lowering secretion of aqueous humour by inhibiting carbonic anhydrase in the ciliary body. These may be divided into two types:
- Systemic, e.g., Acetazolamide, Dichlorphenamide, Ethoxzolamide.
- Topical, e.g., Dorzolamide

Mechanism of Action

(a) During formation of aqueous, both bicarbonate and sodium are actively secreted in posterior chamber. Carbon anhydrase inhibitors (CAI) depress the enzyme concerned (non-competitive, but reversible antagonism) so that synthesis of bicarbonate ions is hampered. This phenomenon causes marked reduction (in an unknown way) in the transport of bicarbonate sodium and water across the cell membrane resulting in fall in IOP. But for this procedure to occur 99% of carbonic anhydrase must be depressed.

(b) A second hypothesis is that CAI induces general acidosis which also causes fall of IOP. But this is possibly not true as I.V. injection of CAI or topical application of CAI causes fall in IOP before systemic acidosis develops. So, to modify the statement it can be said that CAI induced systemic acidosis adds to fall in IOP (it must be noted that diuretic action of CAI plays no role in fall of IOP). Another interesting phenomenon noted is that CAI stimulates retinal pigment epithelium pump mechanism and this might help in drainage of subretinal and intraretinal fluid accumulation during retinal detachment surgery.

Acetazolamide

It is a sulfonamide derivative (Fig.15.1). Its mechanism of action has already been explained. It causes a drop of approximately 30 to 40% IOP. Usually, it is used as short therapy in management of various types of glaucomas.

The peak action after oral ingestion occurs after two hours (approx) as the duration of action is 6-8 hours. Sustained release preparations are effective for even 18 hours. I.V. injection causes fall in IOP within 20 minutes. Addition of a topical beta blocker reduces IOP up to 50%.

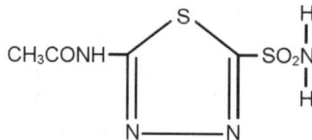

Fig. 15.1. Chemical structure of acetazolamide

Side effects

Side effects include features of G.I. tract irritation, paraesthesia of hand, feet and around mouth, formation of renal stone, lack of libido, disorientation (in hepatic insufficiency patients), disturbances of mode, etc. Periodic blood examination has been recommended in long term use cases. There is risk of bone marrow depression (agranulocytosis, aplastic anaemia, thrombocytopenia, etc.). But such bone marrow depression may be of idiosyncratic type. Usually, potassium loss is insignificant, but still some authorities advocate oral administration of potassium, 1.5 to 2 g/day. Metabolic acidosis may need treatment with sodium bicarbonate and more fluid intake.

Preparation and dosage

Acetazolamide capsules and tablets, 250/500 mg, are available; I.V. preparation contains 500 mg/ vial. Usual oral dose is 125-250 mg, 4 times a day. Sustained release preparations (cap. containing 500 mg) once or twice daily.

Contraindications

- Renal lithiasis cases.
- Severely damaged kidney and liver.
- Idiopathic renal hyperchloremic acidosis.
- Insufficiency of adrenal cortex (as there might be potassium loss).
- Simultaneous use of aspirin should be avoided.

Methazolamide

It is similar in action to acetazolamide but has a less tendency for development of metabolic acidosis and renal stones. Dose is 50-300 mg per day in divided doses.

Dichlorphenamide

Compared to other CAIs, this drug produces more excretion of chloride along with sodium, potassium and bicarbonates. So, there is less chance of metabolic acidosis but potassium loss may be a problem. The usual dose is 25 to 50 mg 1 to 3 times per day orally.

Ethoxzolamide

It is a less potent CAI. The dose is 125 mg, 4 times a day.

Dorzolamide (Topical CAI)

Dorzolamide is an accepted topical CAI. It is available as a 2% solution to be used 2 to 3-times a day. Its mechanism of action is similar to that of other CAIs, but metabolic acidosis does not occur. It is suitable for young people, who suffer from cardiac or respiratory problem. It may act as a good substitute for miotics. It can also be used along with a topical beta-blocker. As it is a sulfonamide derivative, it shares all the side effects of the parent compound. However, its systemic absorption is so less that usually dangerous side effects are not encountered. However, local allergic problems like allergic conjunctivitis, superficial keratopathy and eyelid inflammation are commonly met with.

Brinzolamide

It is another latest topical CAI. It is available as 10 mg/ml eye drop suspension. The dose is B.D. or T.D. It shares all the toxicities of CAIs.

Hyperosmotic Agents

Such agents include chemicals like glycerol, mannitol, ethyl alcohol, ascorbic acid, isosorbide, etc.

Mechanism of Action

These agents increase the osmolarity of the serum; their ocular penetration is very poor and thus by the process of osmosis they reduce the IOP. If the patients are not nauseated, orally effective hyperosmotic agents like glycerol or isosorbide are used, but if they are vomiting (usually they do feel nauseated or may be actually vomiting due to high rise of intraocular pressure), I.V. mannitol is used.

```
        H
        |
   H — C — OH
        |
   H — C — OH
        |
   H — C — OH
        |
        H
```

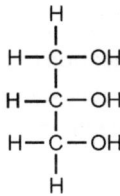

Fig. 15.2. Chemical structure of glycerol

Glycerol

Glycerol (Fig. 15.2) is effective orally; 1 g to 1.5 g/kg of body weight in the form of 50% to 70% solution is usually used. Total dose should not exceed 120 g/ day. Maximum fall of IOP is seen to occur after 1 hr and the duration of effect is usually 5 hours.

Side effects

These include disagreeability due to its nauseating sweet taste, headache, diarrhoea, mental confusion and hyper osmolar coma. It is contraindicated in diabetics, as it is metabolized in the body producing hyperglycaemia.

Mannitol

Mannitol (Fig. 15.3) is given I.V. and is possibly the best drug for quick lowering of IOP (particularly for preparing a patient going for surgery); 5%-20% solutions are available. The dose is 1.5 to 2 g per kg of body weight to be infused very slowly over a period of time extending from 30 to 60 minutes; onset of action is usually prompt (within 30 to 60 minutes) and remains for 6 hours.

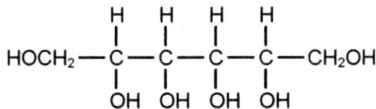

```
                  H    H    H    H
                  |    |    |    |
   HOCH₂ — C — C — C — C — CH₂OH
                  |    |    |    |
                  OH   OH   OH   OH
```

Fig. 15.3. Chemical structure of mannitol

Side effects

These include hypervolemia, pulmonary edema, chest pain, bursting headaches, mental confusion, vomiting, hyponatremia and hypokalemia. Sometimes, urinary retention also occurs due to excessive diuresis. Contraindications of mannitol therapy are renal insufficiency, coronary insufficiency, pulmonary congestion, extreme dehydration and intra cranial haemorrhage.

Ethyl Alcohol

It reduces IOP by following mechanisms:
- Sedative action
- Osmotic effect
- Diuretic effect due to suppression of ADH

Ascorbic Acid

It lowers IOP by following mechanisms:
- Physiologically, concentration of ascorbic acid is 20-40 times higher in aqueous humour than that of serum. If serum concentration of ascorbic acid is elevated more than aqueous concentration, reversal of concentration gradient occurs, leading to marked osmotic effect.
- Acidosis developed due to ascorbic acid therapy stops aqueous production from ciliary epithelium.
- Facility of outflow is also increased.

The usual dose is slow IV infusion (taking about 1 hour) of a solution containing 250 to 500 mg of 20% ascorbic acid.

Isosorbide

It is another orally effective agent. A 45% solution is used; 1 to 2 g/kg of the body weight/ day is usually given in 2 to 4 divided does. Onset of action is usually within 30 min and remains for 5 to 6 hr.

Recent Medications for Glaucoma

These can be divided into three groups:
- Drugs having property of lowering IOP.
- Drugs protecting neural tissue (neuro-protective agents).
- Drugs improving ocular perfusion (vasoactive drugs).

Drugs having Property of Lowering IOP

- Mushroom derivative – Cytochalasin B reduces IOP by improving trabecular outflow.
- Bromocriptine, a potent dopamine agonist (particularly on D2 receptors), reduces IOP by facilitating outflow.
- Some dopamine antagonists like metoclopramide, droperidol, etc., reduce aqueous secretion and improve facility of outflow.
- Ketanserin, a serotonin antagonist, increases outflow facility and reduces IOP.
- Captopril, an ACE inhibitor, reduces IOP by reducing formation of aqueous, improving facility of outflow and increasing uveoscleral outflow.
- Verapamil, a calcium channel blocker, can reduce IOP by increasing trabecular outflow.
- Tetrahydrocortisol, a corticosteroid antagonist, can reduce IOP, particularly in steroid-induced glaucoma cases.
- Vandate, an ATPase inhibitor, reduces aqueous secretion.
- Isobutylmethyl xanthine, a phosphodiestrase inhibitor, inhibits aqueous production.
- Valinomycin, a cyclic peptide and bunazosin, an alpha-1 adrenergic antagonist, can reduce IOP by increasing uveoscleral outflow.
- Chondroitinase ABC, a glycosaminoglycan degrading enzyme, reduces IOP by causing lysis of exteacellular matrix of trabecular meshwork (thus increasing facility).
- Candoxatril, an inhibitor of neural endopeptidase, increases plasma atrial natriuretic peptide (A.N.P.) level with a subsequent fall in IOP.

Neuroprotective Drugs

It has been observed that only lowering of IOP does not arrest the field loss in many cases of glaucoma; so, some agents, which may stop destruction of neural tissues as well, are added to the normal regime. Following belong to this group:

- Memantine, a glutamate receptor blocking drug, reduces the rate of ATP synthesis and thus helps to prevent the cellular death.

- Antioxidants also help to arrest the cellular degeneration.
- Other approaches include induction of heat shock proteins and suppression of nitric oxide synthase; these are also of promising value.
- Other neuroprotective agents under trial are diphenylhydantoin, citicoline, flunarizine, lazaroids, etc.

Drugs Improving Ocular Perfusion (Vasoactive Drugs)

In the management of glaucoma, blood flow of optic nerve head is also very important. Drugs under trial in this group are:

- L-arginine
- Magnesium ions
- Calcium channel blockers

These have been found to improve ocular perfusion.

Drugs used during Glaucoma Surgery

Antifibroblastic agents like 5-FU and Mitomycin C are used in trabeculectomy operation. Other drugs in this group include daunorubicin, bleomycin, cytarabine, doxorubicin, etc. Beta aminopropionitrile and d-penicillamine are used as adjuvant therapy in glaucoma surgery. They inhibit collagen synthesis by subconjunctival fibroblasts. Further, newer drugs include ritidrine, prostaglandin inhibitors, colchicines, etc. (they prevent fibroblastic migration) and triton-A 100, glycerol, etc. (these drugs prevent contraction of scar tissues in the surgical wounds).

CHAPTER 16

Local Anaesthesia in Ophthalmology

Local Anaesthetics

Local anaesthetics are agents which produce reversible block of nerve conduction without any structural damage to the neuron concerned and without any loss of consciousness.

Classification

Local anaesthetics are of two types:
- Ester type, e.g., cocaine, tetracaine, procaine, benzocaine, etc.
- Amide type, e.g., lidocaine, bupivacaine, prilocaine, dibucaine, etc.

The linkage between aromatic moiety and side chain is either by ester bond or amide bond.

Mechanism of Action

Local anaesthetics reduce the permeability of cell membrane to sodium ions and thus they prevent the generation and conduction of nerve impulse.
- Small nerve fibres are more readily affected than large nerve fibres.
- Nonmyelinated nerve fibres are blocked more easily than myelinated nerve fibres.

Commonly Used Local Anaesthetics in Ophthalmic Practice

Following local anaesthetics are commonly used in ophthalmic practice:

- Lidocaine, 1 to 4% (Fig. 16.1)
- Bupivacaine, 0.25 to 0.75%
- Etidocaine, 1 to 1.5%
- Prilocaine, 1 to 2%
- Mepivacaine, 1 to 2%
- Hexylcaine, 1 to 2%
- Proparacaine, 0.75%
- Tetracaine, 0.5%

Common topical anaesthetics

- Lignocaine, 2%, 4%
- Tetracaine, 0.5%
- Proparacaine, 0.75%

Common regional anaesthetics

- Lignocaine, 1 to 2%
- Bupivacaine, 0.5%
- Hexylcaine, 1 to 2%

Commonly Used Drugs along with Local Anaesthetics

Adrenaline and hyaluronidase are two such common drugs. Adrenaline is used to prolong the effect of local anaesthetics and to reduce the toxicity by reducing the absorption from local area.

Hyaluronidase is an enzyme which causes depolymerization of hyaluronic acid (a mucopolysaccharide present in interstitial tissue

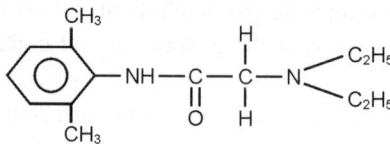

Fig. 16.1. Chemical structure of lidocaine

space) leading to increase in the permeability of the injected fluid. Return of permeability to normal value takes about 24-48 hours.

Strength of hyaluronidase is measured in Turbidity Reducing Units (TRU) and as little as 7 TRU/ml is sufficient to dissolve hyaluronic acid barrier. In addition, a little mechanical pressure on globe (eye) facilitates its spread.

Problems of using adrenaline along with local anaesthetics

Adrenaline is a very risky drug. It can produce high systemic blood pressure and arrhythmia in some individuals. Adrenaline causes delay in wound healing, tissue necrosis and edema formation. These effects are due to the fact that adrenaline increases O_2 demand of local tissues, but as there is associated vasoconstriction, hypoxia results leading to local tissue damage which may even cause local tissue gangrene.

Metabolism of Local Anaesthetics

- Ester type local anaesthetics are metabolized by pseudocholinesterase.
- Amide type local anaesthetics are metabolized by hepatic microsomal enzymes and the enzyme amidase.

Side Effects

Cardio vascular side effects: Mainly depression of heart and this effect is the basis of utilization of procainamide in cardiology. Other CVS side effects include bradycardia, hypotension, cardiac arrhythmias, etc.

CNS side effects: Sudden rapid absorption may produce restlessness, tremor and convulsions. Convulsions are very dangerous as these are often followed by respiratory depression ending in death. The convulsions can be blocked by I.V. diazepam or thiopentone sodium. Sometimes, neuromuscular blockers like suxamethonium aided by artificial respiration are essential to save the life. So, a well equipped emergency tackling set-up should always be ready while using local anaesthetics.

Anaphylactic reaction: It is more common with ester type of local anaesthetics. Milder allergic reactions include asthma, dermatitis, skin rash, etc.

Local tissue damage: Details have already been discussed earlier in this chapter.

Corneal change: Very rarely, corneal change may occur, which is reversible.

Routes of Application

Surface anaesthesia: It is a very popular method in ophthalmic practice. Lignocaine (4% or 2%) has been used, but is now being replaced by proparacaine (0.5%, drops), tetracaine (0.5-2%, drops) and benoxinate (0.4%, drops). Details of drugs used for this purpose have already been discussed. Apart from ophthalmology, surface anaesthetics are used in ENT, urology and gastroenterology.

Infiltration anaesthesia: It is also a very popular method in ophthalmology and details of medicines used has already been discussed. Now-a-days, old facial and retrobulbar blocks have been replaced by peribulbar block.

Nerve block anaesthesia: Retrobulbar block and facial blocks are still being practised by many surgeons.

Other types of anaesthesia: These include spinal anaesthesia, epidural anaesthesia, regional intravenous anaesthesia and field block anaesthesia.

Some Important Local Anaesthetics

Tetracaine (Amethocaine)

It is a popular topical anaesthetic (0.5%) in ophthalmic practice. Onset of action is within 30 seconds and duration lasts up to 20 minutes. Side effects are stinging sensation, punctate epithelial keatopathy, drug allergy, etc.

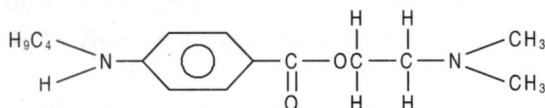

Fig. 16.2. Chemical structure of tetracaine

Proparacaine

It is used as a topical anaesthetic. Usually, 0.75% solution is used. Onset of its effect is within 13 seconds and duration is up to 20 minutes. Corneal toxicity is very rare.

Cocaine

It is no more in use nowadays because of its corneal toxicity, sympathomimetic property and addicting nature. However, it has historical importance as it was the first local anaesthetic obtained from the leaves of a plant Erythroxylon Coca. It was used as 2% solution.

Procaine

It is again a historically important drug as it was the first synthetic local anaesthetic used. It was used as a small area infiltration anaesthetic and spinal anaesthetic but its popularity gradually declined after introduction of lignocaine. Procaine is hydrolyzed in liver and plasma and on hydrolysis it yields PABA which can antagonize the effect of sulfonamide (if concurrently used as antibacterial agent). A 2% injection is the usual preparation.

Lignocaine

It is currently the most used drug and is known as an all purpose anaesthetic. In ophthalmology, 4% (topical) and 2% (infiltration) solutions are commonly used. Its toxicities have been discussed in detail earlier. It is also used I.V. in prophylaxis and treatment of ventricular arrhythmias.

Bupivacaine

Bupivacaine (Fig. 16.3) is a synthetic local anaesthetic, like lignocaine. Onset of its action is slow and unpredictable, but once the anaesthesia occurs, both global anaesthesia and akinesia persist for a longer duration. A 0.75% solution of bupivacaine produces anaestheisa and akinesia for 8 to 12 hours. In ophthalmic practice, usually a combination of 2% lignocaine, 0.75% bupivacaine and 7.5 TRU of

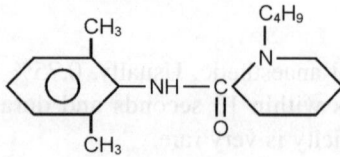

Fig. 16.3. Chemical structure of bupivacaine

hyaluronidase is used for periocular injection, and surgery of any kind may be performed on such type of anaesthetized eye.

Another popular use of bupivacaine is in obstetrics practice where an epidural anaesthesia of 0.5% helps to induce painless delivery due to sensory block without significant involvement of motor functions. But there is a risk of development of ventricular tachycardia and cardiac depression.

CHAPTER **17**

General Anaesthesia in Ophthalmology

General Anaesthetics

General anaesthetics produce reversible loss of consciousness. They abolish pain sensation, produce muscle relaxation and loss of reflexes. They may be in gaseous form or liquid form or I.V. injectible form. They are sometimes used in ophthalmology practice.

Indications

- Examination and operation of children.
- Non co-operative psychotic or deaf adult individuals.
- Apprehensive patients.

Complications

- Oculo-cardiac reflex.
- Expulsive haemorrhage.
- Post-operative vomiting and cough.
- Disorientation of time and space.

Most of these complications can be avoided by proper preanaesthetic medication and by choosing proper anaesthetic agent.

Common General Anaesthetics used in Ophthalmology

At present the most widely used anaesthetic agent is a combination of halothane, N_2O and O_2. Halothane (Fig.17.1) is a pleasant smelling, quick acting, non-irritant, and non-inflammable liquid. Its only deficiencies are poor muscle relaxation and poor analgesia, which are compensated by N_2O and a muscle relaxant.

$$\begin{array}{ccc} & F & H \\ & | & | \\ F - & C - & C - Br \\ & | & | \\ & F & Cl \end{array}$$

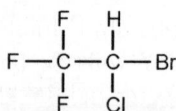

Fig. 17.1. Chemical structure of halothane

The drawbacks of halothane are sensitization of heart to adrenaline (leading to arrhythmias), respiratory depressions, etc. Two more important side effects are development of hepatitis in susceptible individuals and development of a condition called malignant hyperthermia, which occurs rarely. It is genetically determined. There is release of Ca^{2+} from sarcoplasmic reticulum leading to persistent muscle contraction and excessive heat production. Use of succinylcholine may aggravate the condition. The treatment consists of removal of patient to air conditioned chamber, O_2 inhalation, slow I.V. infusion of bicarbonate and I.V. dantrolene, 1 mg per kg (therapy may be repeated as per need).

During retinal detachment surgery, where intravitreal gas is supposed to be given, N_2O administration should be stopped at least 20 minutes prior to administration of gas; otherwise later on there may be shrinkage of gas bubble.

Now-a-days, the anaesthetic agent most widely used in developed countries is isoflurane (Fig. 17.2). The depth of anaesthesia can be adjusted to the desired level and there is no occurrence of seizures with it (hence, it is suitable in neurological cases). Also, there is no sensitization of heart to arrythmogenic action of adrenaline. But it is a very costly drug.

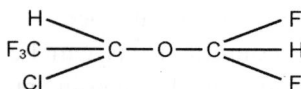

$$\begin{array}{ccccc} H & & & & F \\ & \diagdown & & & \diagup \\ F_3C & = & C - O - C & = & H \\ & \diagup & & & \diagdown \\ Cl & & & & F \end{array}$$

Fig. 17.2. Chemical structure of isoflurane

Peripherally-acting Muscle Relaxants used along with GA in Ocular Surgery

Common agents used are vecuronium and atracurium, which are intermediate acting competitive (non-depolarizing) blocking, peripherally-acting muscle relaxants. Vecuronium is a synthetic drug having shorter duration of action due to its speedy rate of distribution and metabolism. Neostigmine reversal is not usually required unless many repeated doses have been used. As there is no histamine release and ganglionic blockade, cardiovascular stability is good. However, there may be tachycardia in isolated cases.

Atracurium is eliminated by Hofmann elimination plus metabolic degradation by cholinesterases. And so its duration remains unaltered in patients with liver/kidney damage and hypodynamic circulation. Histamine release may occur.

Pre-anaesthetic Medications

Pre-anaesthetic medications have revolutionized anaesthesiology by dramatically reducing complications of general anaesthesia. They not only decrease natural anxiety of the patient due to operation but also prevent complications like aspiration pneumonia. Commonly used drugs in preanaesthetic medications are antiemetics, anxiolytic agents, anticholinergics, H_2 blockers, etc.

Antiemetics

Metoclopramide

Metoclopramide, 10 to 20 mg I.M., is given at least one hour prior to anaesthesia to reduce post-operative vomiting. It possibly acts by three mechanisms:

1. Antagonism to dopamine by acting through D2 receptors.
2. Stimulation of acetyl choline release by myenteric neurons.
3. Antagonism of 5HT by acting through 5-HT3 receptors.

If there is extrapyramidal side effect, diphenhydramine should be used to counteract it.

Alternatively domperidone – a D2 antagonist -- is a better drug as it does not produce any extrapyramidal side effect. The usual dose is 10-40 mg given orally.

The most modern drug in this series is ondansetron which acts by blocking the 5-HT3 receptors in brain and periphery. The usual dose is 8 mg given orally one hour prior to anaesthesia and then two more doses are required, 8 mg each at 8 hourly intervals.

Anxiolytic Agents

The best in this category is lorazepam; it should be used as I.M. injection – 2 mg. It is a good tranquillizer and produces marked amnesia regarding perioperative events.

Cholinergic Blocking Agents

These are especially important to prevent oculocaridac reflex. Atropine sulphate, 0.6 mg I.M., or glycopyrrolate 0.1 to 0.3 mg I.M. is generally used. Glycopyrrolate is a long acting quaternary atropine substitute having no central effect.

H2 Blockers

Classically, ranitidine (150 mg) is used on the night before and on the morning of operation. It reduces gastric acidity (lessening chances of development of stress ulcer) and also reduces volume of gastric content (reducing chance of regurgitation).

CHAPTER 18

Histamine, Histamine Antagonists, Mast Cell Stabilizers and Ocular Decongestants

Histamine

A physiologically active amine, histamine (Fig. 18.1) is found in plant and animal tissue. It is released from mast cells as part of an allergic reaction. Histamine is one of the most important and most widely present alkaloids in human body. It is secreted by almost all the organ systems and plays vital roles in different systems. It is the most important mediator of inflammation and acts as a "double edged sword" – causing protection as well as tissue damage. Histamine antagonists occupy an important place in clinical pharmacology.

Pathophysiological Role of Histamine

Histamine has diverse pathophysiological role like:
- Role as transmitter: In sensory nerve endings, it is believed to play a role in initiation of pain and itching sensation. In central nervous system, it plays many important roles. For example, in hypothalamus and mid brain it helps to regulate body temperature, thirst sensation, cardiovascular function, regulation of release of hormone from anterior pituitary, etc.

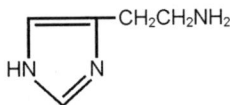

CH₂CH₂NH₂ — HN N

Fig. 18.1. Chemical structure of histamine

- It plays a vital role in gastric secretion.
- It plays an important role in allergic conditions like broncho-constriction, anaphylactic shock, urticaria, angioneurotic edema, etc.
- During an inflammatory process, it is involved in vasodilatation and microcirculation regulation.
- It plays an important role in headache and tissue growth and repair.

Histaminergic Receptors

Three types of histamine receptors have been identified till date: H1, H2 and H3.

H1 receptors: They are present in smooth muscles. Histamine acts on them and causes contraction of gut, bronchoconstriction, contraction of smooth muscles of blood vessels.

H2 receptors: They are present in gastric glands, blood vessels, heart, uterus, etc., and on stimulation cause increased gastric secretion, vasodilatation (due to effect on smooth muscles of blood vessels), stimulation of heart, relaxation of uterus (observed in rats), etc.

H3 receptors: They are present in CNS. Detailed functions of these receptors are not yet known.

Histamine Antagonists

Histamine antagonists can be divided into two broad groups: H1 blockers and H2 blockers.

H1 Blockers

(a) First generation: These have CNS depressant property together with anticholinergic effect. Important members of this group are chlorpheniramine, diphenhydramine, promethazine, meclizine, cyclizine, etc.

(b) Second generation: These are practically free from sedative and anticholinergic effects. But some people do experience such effects. The important members of this group are astemizole, terfenadine, cetrizine, loratadine, fexofenadine, etc.

(C) Miscellaneous agents: Some drugs may either suppress the production or release of endogenous histamine, thereby exhibiting antihistamine effect. Examples of such drugs include epinephrine, mast cell stabilizing drugs and even theophylline.

Mechanism of action of H1 blockers

Most of them act by competitive antagonism with histamine of receptor site. For example, cetirizine can inhibit migration of inflammatory cells, particularly eosinophils. It also inhibits mast cell degranulation. Loratadine, in addition to antihistamine effect, possesses a direct effect on mast cells. Cetirizine and loratadine both inhibit platelet activating factor which is supposed to be an important mediator during acute inflammatory conditions.

Therapeutic uses of antihistaminics (H1 blockers)

(a) *Topical use*: They are used in allergic conjunctivitis, atopic and giant papillary conjunctivitis, vernal keratoconjunctivitis, etc. Many a times, antihistaminics need combined use with corticosteroids, prostaglandin synthase inhibitors and mast cell stabilizers.

(b) *Systemic use*:
- Atopic and contact dermatitis
- Hay fever
- Allergic rhinitis
- Motion sickness and vertigo (e.g. diphenhydramine)
- Parkinsonism (drug-induced) (e.g. diphenhydramine)
- Pre-anaesthetic medication, particularly in children (e.g. promethazine)
- Atitussive (e.g. chlorpheniramine)
- To control cancer chemotherapy induced vomiting (e.g. promethazine).

Side effects

Milder side effects are sedation and atropine-like effect. The dangerous side effect of terfenadine and astemizole are polymorphic, ventricular tachycardia. That is why erythromycin, clarithromycin, ketoconazole, itraconazole, etc., must not be used with these drugs as they can precipitate cardiac arrhythmia (Torsades de pointes). Azythromycin and fluconazole are relatively safer drugs in this respect.

Contraindications

- Dry eye syndromes (as antihistamines diminish tear secretion).
- Contact lens users.
- Patient allergic to drug molecule itself.
- First trimester of pregnancy.
- Narrow angle glaucoma.
- Prostatic hypertrophy.

Some important topical H1 blockers

- Chlorpheniramine, 0.3%
- Dexbrompheniramine, 0.3%
- Pyrilamine, 0.1%
- Levocabastine, 0.05%

Common Systemic H1 Blockers used in Ophthalmic Practice

Pheniramine maleate

It (Fig. 18.2) is the most popular, oldest and widely used anti-allergic drug. Its dose is 25-50 mg twice daily. In children the dose is: 4-12 months –7.5 mg twice daily;1-5 yr, –15 mg twice daily; 6-14 yr, –15 mg-22.5 mg twice daily.

It produces sedative effect, dry mouth, G.I. disturbance, etc. Blood dyscrasias have been reported in some cases. It should always

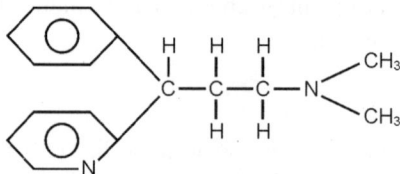

Fig. 18.2. Chemical structure of pheniramine

be used with caution in narrow angle glaucoma subjects, prostatic hypertrophic males and lactating mothers.

Diphenhydramine

It (Fig. 18.3) is also a popular antiallergic of past. Its dose in adults is 25 to 50 mg daily. In children, the dose is to be adjusted accordingly, it but should not be used in children below 6 years. It should also be avoided during pregnancy and lactation. Its side effects are mainly sedation and anticholinergic effect.

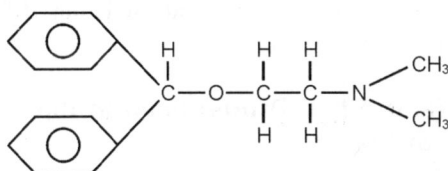

Fig. 18.3. Chemical structure of diphenhydramine

Promethazine

Promethazine (Fig. 18.4) is yet another antiallergic of the past. Its dose for adults is 10-20 mg 2 to 3 times daily. In children, the dose is adjusted accordingly

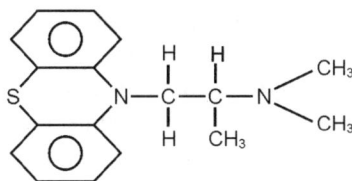

Fig. 18.4. Chemical structure of promethazine

Its side effects are similar to those for pheniramine maleate. It is to be avoided in children below 12 years, phenothiazine-induced jaundice cases, epilepsy, narrow angle glaucoma, hypertensive crisis, prostatic hypertrophy, hepatic insufficiency, impaired respiratory function, etc.

Terfenadine

It was a very popular second generation anti-allergic drug, but its popularity has declined nowadays due to its cardiac toxicity which has already been discussed. The usual dose is 60 mg twice or 120 mg once per day. It is contraindicated in children below 3 years.

Cetirizine

It is most popular and widely used drug presently. Its dose is 10 mg once per day. It is to be avoided in children below 6 years, pregnancy and lactation. Its common side effects are sedation, dry mouth, G.I. tract irritation, agitation, headache, etc.

H1 Blockers (and Allied Drugs) used In the Management of Vertigo

(a) *Drugs which suppress the labyrinthine apparatus*: These agents either suppress the receptor cells or suppress the central cholinergic pathway in vestibular nucleus. These drugs are classified as follows:
- H1 receptor blocker possessing anticholinergic effect, e.g., dimenhydrinate, diphenhydramine, promethazine, cyclizine, cinnarizine, etc.
- Pure anticholinergic drugs like atropine, hyoscine, etc.
- Phenothiazine derivatives possessing antiemetic property, e.g., prochlorperazine.

(b) *Diuretics*: These agents act by reducing the labyrinthine fluid pressure, e.g., frusemide, thiazide, etc.

(c) *Antianxiety compounds and antidepressants*: These agents modify the sensation of vertigo, e.g., amitryptaline, diazepam.

(d) *Vasodilating agents*: Agents which improve the flow of blood in labyrinth and brain stem are found to reduce vertigo, e.g., betahistine, nicotinic acid, naftidrofuryl.

(e) *Corticosteroids*: Steroids are particularly useful in cases of intralabyrinthine edema due to viral infections and other reasons.

H2 Receptors Blockers

These drugs are used in reduction of gastric acidity and have no ophthalmic indications as yet.

Mast Cell Stabilizers

Mechanism of Action

During an allergic process when an antigen binds to two adjacent IgE molecules on the surface of mast cells, there occurs an increased inflow of calcium ions inside the cell and the secretion of various substances of mast cells starts, which are kept stored normally within numerous granules present inside the cell. All these substances (histamine, serotonin, leukotrienes, SRS-A, PG, an eosinophil chemotactic factor, heparin, etc.) are able to produce violent inflammatory response. It has been found that high level of cyclic guanosine monophosphate (CGMP) bears a negative feed back effect on release of inflammatory materials from mast cells.

Commonly Used Mast Cell Stabilizers

- Sodium cromoglycate (also called cromolyn sodium).
- Ketotifen.
- Miscellaneous drugs: Oxatomide, olopatadine, cetirizine human IgE pentapeptide, nedocromil, zinc, Iodoxamide, etc.

Sodium cromoglycate (Fig. 18.5)

It is poorly absorbed from gut. It is used as inhaler (for bronchial asthma), nasal spray and eye drop. Its exact mechanism of action is not yet known. However, it is believed that sodium cromoglycate inhibits cyclic nucleotide phosphodiesterase. This phenomenon causes increase in cellular level of CGMP dependent protein kinase leading to phosphorylation of membrane bound cell protein of mast cells. This phenomenon is called stabilization of mast cell (which is essential for degranulation). In addition to this, sodium chromoglycate suppresses activation of eosinophils, monocytes and neutrophils. However, it does not interfere with binding or interaction of antigen to cell surface IgE.

It has no bronchodilator property and so it is of no use during an acute attack of asthma. In ophthalmology, 2% solution is used in vernal conjunctivitis, other allergic types of conjunctivitis, contact lens induced giant papillary conjunctivitis and to some extent in ligneous

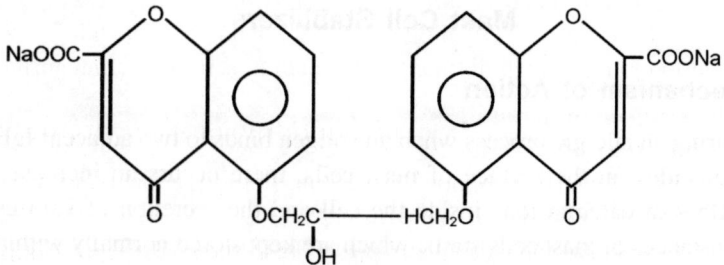

Fig. 18.5. Chemical structure of cromolyn sodium

conjunctivitis. Sometimes, the drug molecule itself may show allergic reaction. Otherwise, as such it is a compound remarkably free from side effects.

Ketotifen

It is basically a H1 blocker antihistamine. It is well absorbed orally. Its dose is 1 to 2 mg BD for adults and 0.5 mg BD for children. It works by antagonizing calcium (whose intracellular high concentration is so important for degranulation). In addition it antagonizes SRS-A.

Lodoxamide

It is a mast cell stabilizer 2500 times superior to sodium cromoglycatye in potency. It is available as 0.1% solution.

Human IgE pentapeptide

It is a pentapeptide, which has been found to obstruct immediate wheal and flare response. The exact mechanism of action is not yet well understood. However, suggestions are that it may prevent binding of IgE to mast cell receptors or it may antagonize substance P. In allergic conjunctivitis, 0.5% solution produces very good response.

Commonly used Ocular Decongestants

Following are the commonly used ocular decogestants:
- Phenylephrine, 0.08% to 0.2%.
- Tetrahydrozoline, 0.01% to 0.05%.
- Oxymetazoline, 0.01% to 0.05%.

- Xylometazoline, 0.1% (Fig. 18.6).
- Naphazoline, 0.01% to 0.1% (Fig. 18.7).
- Tramazoline, 0.05% to 0.1%.

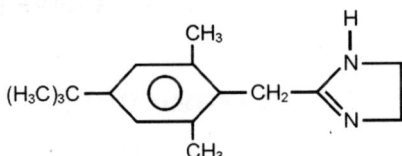

Fig. 18.6. Chemical structure of xylometazoline

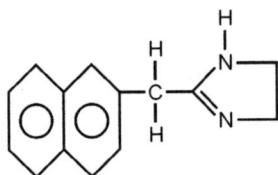

Fig. 18.7. Chemical structure of naphazoline

Mechanism of action

These agents are basically vasoconstrictors and act by stimulating alpha adrenergic receptors. In ophthalmology, they are usually used to get relief from conjunctival hyperaemia and also from low degree edema. They are also used as nasal decongestants prior to lacrimal apparatus surgery.

Contraindications

These agents are contraindicated in hypertension, diabetes mellitus, cardiac disease, hyperthyroidism, dry eyes, dry nose, narrow angle glaucoma, (particularly phenylephrine which causes dilatation of pupil over 0.125%) and in children below 2 years.

Side effects

Important side effects include sudden dilatation of pupil precipitating acute attack of narrow angle glaucoma, headache, angina pain, high blood pressure, development of chronic follicular conjunctivitis (and also allergic type of blepharoconjunctivitis), etc.

CHAPTER 19

Some Important Pharmacological Agents Used in Ocular Therapeutics

Vasodilators

The most popular drug in this group is pentoxiphylline. Others are cyclanadelate, xantinol nicotinate, calcium channel blockers like nifedipine, etc.

Pentoxiphylline

It is a derivative of theophylline (belonging to methyl xanthine group). It improves microcirculation of ischaemic area by improving flexibility of RBC and by reducing the viscosity of blood. Side effects like G.I. irritation may occur. The usual dose is 400 mg BD to TD. In ophthalmology, it is used in occlusive retinal vascular diseases. Other indications are transient ischaemic attacks, peripheral vascular diseases, etc. It is used in males for treating infertility due to lack in motility of sperms.

Cyclandelate

It is another popular drug which produces its effect by relaxing smooth muscles (similar to papaverine). The usual dose is 200-400 mg TDS.

Xantinol Nicotinate

It is made up of xanthine plus nicotinic acid; it increases blood flow. The usual dose is 300-600 mg TDS orally.

Isoxuprine

It is a beta adrenergic receptor agonist which also relaxes the smooth muscles. The usual oral dose is 20 mg OD after food.

Tolazoline

Tolazoline (Fig.19.1) is an alpha adrenergic receptor antagonist. It is given by retrobulbar route-10 mg/ day × 2 weeks, produces beneficial vasodilator effect.

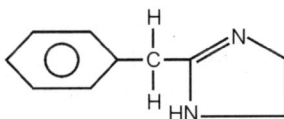

Fig. 19.1. Chemical structure of tolazoline

Calcium Channel Blockers and Angiotensin Converting Enzyme Inhibitors

Calcium channel blockers like nifedipine and angiotensin converting enzyme inhibitors like captopril have been tried with good results in patients having occasional vascular spasm.

Drugs Used to Control Haemorrhage

Antifibrinolytic Agents

To this group belong tranexamic acid and aminocaproic acid. They act by inhibiting plasminogen activators and also to some extent by inhibiting the effect of plasmin on fibrin leading to inhibition of lysis of a fibrin clot. These agents are used in cases of hyphema to reduce the risk of secondary haemorrhage. They are also used as preventive measures to reduce the incidence of intraoperative and postoperative haemorrhages. Their side effects are minor like vertigo, fall in BP, nausea, etc. They should be avoided during pregnancy and in the patients with suspected intravascular coagulopathy. The usual dose of tranexamic acid is 0.5 to 1 g TD × 3-5 days. The usual dose of aminocaproic acid is 50 mg/kg every 4 hours, not exceeding a dose of 30 g/day. It is also available for topical use containing 30% aminocaproic acid in 2% carboxy-polymethylene.

Ethamsylate

It prevents haemorrhage from small blood vessels during surgical procedures or even as such by inhibiting prostacycline synthetase. This leads to prevention of prostacycline induced vasodilatation and antiplatelet aggregation. The oral dose is 500 mg every 4 to 6 hours till bleeding is controlled. For prophylactic purpose, 1 to 2 ampoules (each amp. containing 250 mg/2 ml) are given I.V., one hour prior to surgery. Side effects are minor like headache, skin rash, etc. The agent has been tried with success in cataract operation.

Calcium Dobesilate

It has been tried in diabetic retinopathy. It retards the breakdown of collagen and reduces viscosity of blood thus improving blood flow. The usual dose is 500 mg to 1 g per day × 4-6 months in divided doses, followed by 500 mg/day. Side effects are minor.

Vitamin K

It is needed in individuals with deficient vitamin. K in blood, as in cases of hepatic diseases, prolonged antimicrobial therapy, obstructive jaundice, etc. The usual dose is:
- Menapthone: 5-20 mg/day.
- Menadione: 5-10 mg TD/day.

Adrenochrome Monosemicarbazone

It reduces capillary fragility, reduces oozing from surface and prevents microvessel bleeding (e.g. retinal haemorrhage, epistaxis, haematuria, etc.). The usual dose is 1.5 mg given orally or I.M.

Rutin

It is a plant glycoside which reduces capillary bleeding. It is found to be effective (20-30 mg BD to TD orally) along with Vitamin C (50 to 100 mg).

Conjugated Estrogen

This agent is found to be useful in diabetic retinopathy and it also prevents surgical or traumatic bleeding. It possibly acts by preventing capillary permeability. The usual dose is 20 mg I.M./I.V. given 6 to 12 hourly.

Thrombin

This enzyme, if added intermittently to irrigation fluid (100 IU/ml) during vitrectomy, reduces chance of bleeding, particularly while cutting vascularised preretinal membranes. However, acute intraocular inflammation has been reported. This agent has also been used in anterior segment surgery, but endothelial damage may be a problem.

Botropase

It is an aqueous solution of haemocoagulase prepared from the venom of Bothrops jararaca or B. atorox and is used (usual dose for adults 1 ml, I.M., SOS) to prevent haemorrhage during surgical procedures.

Aprotinin

It is a naturally occurring proteolytic enzyme which inhibits plasmin and kallikrein resulting in inhibition of fibrinolysis and the incidence of blood loss during surgery is minimized.

Antiviscosity Agents

An increase in blood viscosity has been suspected to play an important role in the genesis of various ocular conditions like ischaemic optic neuropathy, normotensive glaucoma, macular degeneration, retinopathy associated with venous stasis and diabetes. Various methods adopted to counteract such hyperviscosity states include:

- Plasmapheresis, a technique by which high molecular weight plasma proteins are reduced.
- Use of hypolipidemic drugs.
- Hemodilution, wherein blood corpuscular elements are reduced.

• Use of drugs which inhibit platelet aggregation, increase fibrinolysis and decrease coagulability of blood.

Thrombolytic and Fibrinolytic Agents

The ophthalmic clinical conditions where these agents are used are central retinal artery or vein occlusion, management of hyphaema, glaucoma surgery for obtaining postoperative fibrinolysis during vitretomy to prevent post-vitrectomy fibrin formation during macular surgery, etc. Such agents are:

Streptokinase and Urokinase

Streptokinase is obtained from hemolytic streptococci and urokinase from cultures of human renal cells. These agents activate plasminogen to plasmin which in turn causes lysis of insoluble fibrin clot into smaller units of soluble fractions. Of the two, streptokinase is more antigenic than urokinase. Streptokinase can be given 600, 000 IU as loading dose I.V. followed by 200,000 and 50 thousand IU at 8 hourly intervals. The solution used for I.V. can be used in anterior chamber (1000 IU). It can also be used in vitreous chamber (2000 IU).

Urokinase is used as 6000 IU/kg I.V. as initial dose. The same dose is repeated as infusion over 12 hours. Anterior chamber dose is 2500 IU. Both the drugs are contraindicated if there is any recent history of internal haemorrhage (within two months) and cardiovascular accident. These should also be avoided in cases of brain tumour and aneurysms. Fever and hypersensitive reactions are very common as side effects. Corneal toxicity following intraocular administration has also been reported.

Recombinant Tissue Plasminogen Activator (rt – PA)

It is also called alteplase. It is produced from human tissue culture by recombinant DNA technology. It is more specific in the sense that it activates only that plasminogen which is bound to fibrin clot and has practically no action on circulating plasminogen. The compound is non-antigenic. However, fever, nausea, etc., may occur. I.V. dose is 50 to 100 mg. Intracameral dose is 4 to 6 microgram and intravitreal dose is 5 to 25 microgram.

Arvin

It is an enzyme obtained from the venom of a viper. Agkistroden rhodostoma is also a fibrinolytic agent which is particularly useful in venous thrombosis. I.V. infusion 2 to 3 units per kg for 6 to 8 hours reduces the fibrinogen level quickly and a maintenance dose of 2 units per kg body wt. is used I.V. every 12 hours. In case of an overdose, a specific antivenom antidote is also available. Compared to conventional anticoagulants it has a lesser tendency of bleeding manifestations.

Miscellaneous compounds which are under trial are acylated plasminogen streptokinase activator (APSAC) complex and recombinant single chain urokinase plasminogen activator.

Anticoagulants

The main anticoagulants used in ophthalmology are heparin, oral anticoagulants and certain agents like prostaglandin synthesis inhibitors.

Heparin

Mechanism of action

It acts by activating plasma antithrombin III. Then the complex gets bound to clotting factors of intrinsic and common pathways like Xa, IIa, IXa, XIa, XIIa and XIIIa and the factors get inactivated. But factor VIIa involved in extrinsic pathway is not affected. The anticoagulant action is due to suppression of conversion of fibrinogen to fibrin operated mainly through inhibition of factor Xa and thrombin.

Other actions of heparin include:

- Clearance of post-prandial lipemic plasma.
- Antiplatelet function.
- Suppressant effect on collagen polymerization, cellular proliferation and contraction.
- It is also claimed to possess antiherpetic effect and retardation effect on ocular growth factors.

Use in ophthalmology

- Central retinal artery or vein occlusion.

- Management of corneal ulcers, filamentary keratopathy ischaemic scleral and peripheral corneal diseases, etc.
- For treatment of haematomas (applied as ointment).
- It has also been used in irrigation fluid during intraocular surgery to decrease intraocular fibrin.
- Used in low doses as a prophylactic agent to prevent deep vein thrombosis in post operative cases.

Other important therapeutic indications

- Its most important use is to prevent pulmonary embolism.
- It is used in vascular surgery, haemodialysis and in cases of prosthetic heart valves.

Dosage

- It can be given as I.V. bolus dose – 5 thousand to 10 thousand IU – 4 to 6 hourly. Alternatively, the initial bolus may be followed by continuous I.V. drip 750-1000 IU/hour. Control of dose is monitored by activated partial thromboplastin time (aPTT) measurement which is maintained either 50 to 80 sec or 1.5 to 2.5 times the pretreatment value of the patient. However, if this test is not possible whole blood clotting time should be measured and it should be kept at least 2 times the normal value.
- The 2nd method is deep subcutaneous injection – 10 thousand to 20 thousand U – 8 to 12 hourly – particularly in cases where continuous I.V. drip is not possible. The onset of action takes about 30 to 60 min after subcutaneous injection.
- Another popular method is called low dose subcutaneous regimen. Here 5 thousand U is injected (SC) – 8 to 12 hourly prior to surgery and is used for 7 to 10 days till the patient is ambulatory to prevent deep vein thrombosis. Incidence of bleeding during surgery is negligible. However, this method is contraindicated during neurosurgery, hip joint or pelvic surgery.

Important side effects

- Haemorrhagic manifestations – usually haematuria.

- Mild thrombocytopenia.
- Hypersensitive reactions.

Relative contraindications

- Severe hypertension, where there is a risk of cerebral haemorrhage.
- Chronic alcoholics and patients receiving aspirin and antiplatelet drugs.
- Blood diseases like haemophilia.
- Recent history of internal haemorrhage (gastric, intracranial, etc.).

LMW heparins (low molecular weight heparins)

These have been recently fractionated from the usual heparin. These have selective inhibitory action on factor Xa and very little action on IIa. These are better absorbed and chances of bleeding are less. They have little effect on a PTT and whole blood clotting time. Indications are the same as that of heparin.

Heparin antagonist

It is protamine sulfate. It neutralizes heparin and is used IV, 1 mg of protamine neutralizes, 100 U of heparin. However, it is rarely used and usually a fresh whole blood transfusion is needed. Protamine is generally needed after cardio-vascular surgery.

Oral Anticoagulants

Drugs of this group act indirectly by restricting the synthesis of vitamin K dependent clotting factors in liver. These drugs act by competitive antagonism with vitamin K interfering with formation of active vitamin K hydroquinone and so there is reduction in the rate of synthesis of clotting factors II, VII, IX and X.

Although the synthesis of the above factors is practically stopped within 2-4 hours of administration of oral anticoagulants, but it takes about 1 to 3 days for therapeutic effect to occur, as during this period the preformed clotting factors decline progressively.

The dose is regulated by repeated measurement of prothrombin time.

Adverse Effects

- Most important effect is bleeding. It may start as haematuria, haemoptysis, epistaxis, bleeding gum, intracranial haemorrhage, gut bleeding from peptic ulcer, etc.
- There may be cutaneous gangrene.
- Other side effects include urticaria, alopecia, teratogenic effect, etc.

Dosage

- Warfarin sodium (Fig. 19.2) – loading dose is 10 to 15 mg. Maintenance dose is 2 to 10 mg per day.
- Bishydroxycoumarin – loading dose is 200 mg x 2 days followed by maintenance dose of 50 to 100 mg per day
- Acenocoumarol – loading dose is 8-12 mg and maintenance dose is 2-8 mg per day.
- Ethyl biscoumacetate – loading dose is 900 mg and maintenance dose is 300-600 per day.

Management of Anticoagulant Induced Bleeding

- The drug has to be stopped.
- Either fresh whole blood or fresh frozen plasma transfusion should be given.

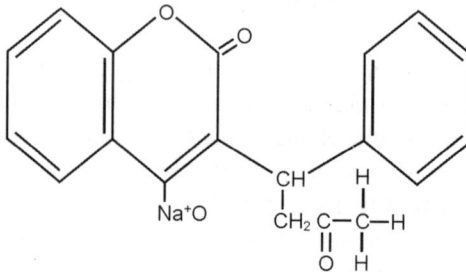

Fig. 19.2. Chemical structure of warfarin sodium

- An effective antidote – phytonadione (vit K1) – should be used. It is relatively quick acting but however, clotting factors resynthesis takes about 6-24 hours time. The dose of vit K1 depends on degree of hypoprothrombinaemia. In severe cases 10 mg IM followed by 5 mg – 4 hourly. In moderate cases 10 mg IM followed by 5 mg once or twice depending on response. In less serious cases only stoppage of few doses of oral anticoagulants is sufficient.

Factors which Influence Activity of Oral Anticoagulants

The activity is increased by:
- Conditions leading to less supply of Vit K to liver, like malabsorption syndrome, malnutrition, etc.
- Hyperthyroidism (due to rapid degradation of clotting factors).
- In hepatic diseases and chronic alcoholism where synthesis of clotting factors is hampered.

The activity is reduced by:
- Warfarin resistance – genetically determined.
- Pregnancy – the clotting factor level of plasma is very high.
- Renal diseases like nephrotic syndrome where the plasma protein containing bound drug is lost in urine.

Contraindications

All contraindications as applied to heparin are applicable here also. In addition, it is totally contraindicated during pregnancy. Given in early pregnancy, Warfarin produces fetal warfarin syndrome characterized by various bony defects like hypoplasia of nose, hand bones, eye socket and general retardation of growth. Given in late pregnancy, it causes damage to CNS, hypoprothrombinemia of fetus and haemorrhagic manifestations in fetus.

Drug interactions

Following drugs increase the anticoagulant activity:
- Drugs like broad spectrum antibiotics depress the gut flora leading to lack of Vit K synthesis.

- Additive action with drugs like newer cephalosporins (Cefoperazone, Cefamandole, etc.), as these drugs also produce hypoprothrombinaemia.
- Drugs inhibiting platelet aggregation like aspirin and dipyridamole increase the chance of bleeding manifestation.
- Phenylbutazone reduces protein binding of Warfarin and also inhibits metabolism of more active S enantiomer (but induction of R enantiomer) as a result of which there is an increased anticoagulant activity.
- Clofibrate, anabolic steroid, quinidine and phenformin potentiate the action of Warfarin.
- Chronic use of liquid paraffin reduces Vit K absorption and, hence, leads to increased activity of Warfarin.
- Phenytoin and tolbutamide produce inhibition of Warfarin metabolism and vice versa.
- Long acting sulfonamides, phenytoin, indomethacin and probenecid group of drugs cause displacement of warfarin from plasma protein binding site and so increased effect of Warfarin occurs.
- Certain drugs like metronidazole, allopurinol, cimetidine, erythromycin, chloramphenicol, etc., retard the metabolism of warfarin and induce more anticoagulant activity.

Following drugs decrease the anticoagulant activity:

- Barbiturates, griseofulvin and rifampicin induce enzymes which increase the metabolism of warfarin and so the dose adjustment has to be done if these drugs are also used concurrently. But after stoppage of these drugs, if the dose of warfarin is not lowered fatal bleeding may occur.
- Oral contraceptives elevate the level of clotting factors in blood and so they reduce the anticoagulant activity of warfarin.

Ophthalmic Indications

Indications are practically same as discussed under heparin therapy. In addition it has also been used in cavernous sinus thrombosis. However, the maximum utility of oral anticoagulants has been found to be in cases of retinal vein occlusion.

Antiplatelet Drugs

Prostaglandin Synthesis Inhibitors

Aspirin

Drugs like aspirin in low dose inhibit synthesis of thromboxane A2 (TXA2). Thromboxane is a strong platelet aggregation stimulator. However, if the dose is increased, prostacycline synthesis is also reduced (prostacycline is a powerful inhibitor of platelet aggregation). So, suppression of blood coagulability is observed to be the maximum with low dose aspirin (60 to 100 mg/ day). The effect of aspirin on platelets is irreversible. The platelets regenerate at a speed of 10% per day and so effect of single day therapy of aspirin lasts for many days.

Aspirin is indicated in the following conditions:

* In prethrombotic states to prevent intravascular thrombosis. It is used in cases of amaurosis fugax, transient ischaemic attacks induced by atherosclerosis of caroid artery and also intracardiac thrombosis.
* Prophylaxis of retinal vein occlusion.
* In diabetic retinopathy cases.

Its side effects include GI tract irritation and it may even lead to bleeding peptic ulcer. Aspirin should always be discontinued at least 3 to 12 days before any surgical treatment to avoid excessive bleeding during surgery. In children, serum transaminase should always be noted, as an increase in their level indicates hepatic damage. Aspirin therapy in children suffering from viral infections like influenza may precipitate hepatic encephalopathy, popularly known as Reye's syndrome.

Dipyridamole

It inhibits phosphodiesterase and increases platelet cAMP by blocking the uptake of adenosine. The result is potentiation of PGI2 and interference with platelet aggregation. However, usually it is used in combination with warfarin, particularly in prosthetic heart valve cases. The dose is 150 mg per day.

Ticlopidine

It is a relatively new drug which acts on fibrinogen receptors situated on platelet membrane. As a result of which fibrinogen is unable to bind to activated platelets leading to inhibition of platelet aggregation and clot retraction. The dose is 250 mg twice daily after meals.

Sedatives

They can be divided into two groups:
- Benzodiazepines
- Non-benzodiazepines

Benzodiazepines

Drugs of this group produce sedative action by potentiation of neural inhibition in central nervous system by GABA. These produce anxiolytic effect, and muscle relaxation. Some of these also possess anticonvulsant action (e.g. diazepam). When used for long term, a type of drug-dependence may develop, which can be overcome by gradual withdrawal.

The common benzodiazepines used along with their doses are listed below:
- Diazepam (Fig. 19.3) – 5 mg at bed time
- Lorazepam – 1 mg at bed time
- Alprazolam – 0.25 mg at bed time
- Chlordiazepoxide – 10 mg at bed time

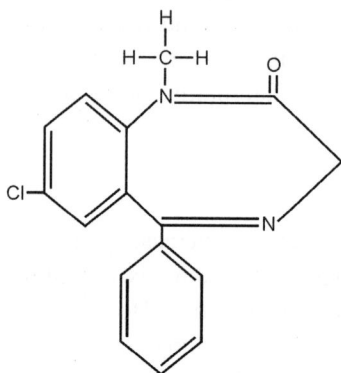

Fig. 19.3. Chemical structure of diazepam

Non-benzodiazepines

Following drugs belong to this group:

- Azopirones, e.g., Buspirone, which acts probably by its selective partial agonistic action on 5HT 1A receptors and a weak dopamine D2 blocking action. It is contraindicated in epilepsy and hepato-renal insufficiency. A dose of 5 mg once or twice a day gives satisfactory results.
- Imidazopyridine derivatives, e.g., Zolpidem. Zolpidem is a recently introduced compound. It possibly selectively binds to omega 1 subtype of BZD receptors and that is why there is no muscle relaxation and anticonvulsant action. A dose of 5 mg at bed time is sufficient for sedative purpose.
- Cyclopyrrolone derivatives, e.g., Zopiclone. Zopiclone is another currently used compound, particularly for weaning off patients addicted to benzodiazepines. It also acts by potentiation of GABA, but binds to a different place than benzodiazepines. A dose of 7.5 mg tablet at bedtime is sufficient.

Anticataractous Substances

Till today no such compound has been found which possesses anticataractous property beyond doubt. But many substances have been claimed to possess such properties and the list is very long. The important compounds belonging to this group are:

- Glutathione.
- Antioxidants like Vit E, Vit. C, Beta carotene, etc.
- Compounds containing inorganic iodine.
- Anti-inflammatory compounds like aspirin, bendazac, flunoxapropen, etc.
- A sulfur containing compound, tiopronin.
- A pantothenic acid derivative, pantetheine.

Pharmacotherapy Related to Lacrimal System

Artificial Tears

While preparing artificial tears certain facts are to be taken into consideration:

- The solution should contain appropriate amount of sodium, potassium, calcium and bicarbonate.
- Ideal pH of ophthalmic solution lies between 7.4 and 7.7.
- Osmolarity of the preparation should be between 200 and 280 mOsm.
- Ideally, it should be preservative-free. However, chlorobutanol 0.5% may be allowed.
- A mucin polymer, which can act as mucin substitute, is used to prolong the effectivity of artificial tears. Compounds used for this purpose are carboxy methylcellulose, hyaluronic acid, chondroitin sulfate, polyvinyl alcohol hydroxypropyl methyl cellulose, hydroxy ethylcellulose, etc. The viscosity of such artificial tear preparations should be between 0.7 and 4.5 centipoise (cps).

Preparations of artificial tears are available in the market in the following forms:

- Drop form
- Ointment form
- Ocusert form
- Gel form—It is a relatively newer preparation where a synthetic polymer of acrylic acid is used which dissolves at a very slow rate keeping the cornea and conjunctiva moist.

Mucolytic Agents

These are usually used in filamentary keratopathy cases to remove the excess of mucous plaques formed. The commonest agent used for the purpose is acetylcysteine (10% to 20% solution). But it is very costly and possesses unpleasant odour. In addition, hyperosmotic sodium chlorides drop (2% to 5%, 4 to 5 times/ day) and hypertonic saline (10% to 20% ointment at bed time) have been found to be effective in filamentary keratopathy cases.

Drugs Stimulating Secretion of Tears

In dry eye syndrome, the tear secretion can be increased by many pharmacological agents. The most popular is bromhexine (8 to 16 mg thrice daily orally), which directly stimulates goblet cells to secrete more mucin. Another popular drug is isobutylmethylxanthine, a phosphodiesterase inhibitor which can be used topically. Other drugs used topically which can stimulate tear production are physalaemine and eledoisin.

Dyes Used Commonly in Ophthalmology

Fluorescein

It is a fluorescent dye, chemically (Fig.19.4) similar to phenolphthalein. It is obtained from the chemical reaction between phthalic acid and resorcinol. The preparation used is fluorescein sodium solution (2% for topical use and 5%, 10% and 20% for internal use). At pH 7.4, maximum yellowish green fluorescence is obtained.

Important topical uses of this dye are:

- Used for staining to detect corneal ulcer and abrasion. Fluorescein solution is liable to get contaminated with Pseudomonas aeruginosa and so a freshly prepared 2% solution should always be used. Alternatively, fluorescein sodium 4% strips can be used for staining purpose.
- Used during applanation tonometry.
- Used to perform Siedel's test to detect any wound leaks.
- Used for the assessment of stability of precorneal tear film by BUT test.
- Testing of naso-lacrimal passage.
- Used in radial keratotomy operation to observe the markings of radial cuts.
- During fitting of hard contact lenses (obsolete nowadays).

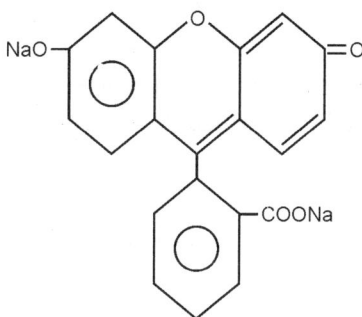

Fig. 19.4. Chemical structure of fluorescein sodium

The dye, on intravenous administration, gets bound to plasma protein and its absorption of light is maximum (absorption peak) between 465 and 490 nm and emission peak is between 520 and 530 nm. The dye can impart fluorescence even at 1 in 1,000,000 dilution, which can be appreciated by using ultra violet light. Elimination via kidney and liver is usually complete within 24 to 36 hours. Usually, 3 ml. of 20% solution is used for intravenous purpose. Common indications of I.V. fluorescein are:

- Fundus fluorescein angiography.
- Study of vascular architecture of iris in conditions like rubeosis iridis, vascular tumours, etc.
- Study of outflow of aqueous humour by fluorescein photometry, etc.

Its side effects are usually negligible. However, hypersensitive reactions, nausea, vomiting, etc., may occur. Anaphylactic reactions are not uncommon.

Indocyanin

Indocyanin is yet another dye, though more toxic than flurescein but gives a clearer picture of ARMD by angiography.

Rose Bengal

Its 1% solution is used to stain devitalized epithelial cells, mucous threads and corneal filaments. It is a painful test as it is performed without any anaesthetic agent. It is usually avoided nowadays. However, it is supposed to be a very sensitive test in evaluating the prognosis of dry eye cases.

Recent Advancements in Pharmacotherapy of ARMD (Age Related Macular Degeneration)

Verteporfin

It is used for photodynamic therapy of ARMD – exudative type associated with choroidal neovascular membrane.

It is injected I.V. and after it reaches choroidal circulation it is light-activated by a nonthermal laser source. Activation in presence of oxygen leads to generation of free radicals which lead to thrombosis, vascular damage, etc., of neovascularizations of choroids. The drug is excreted mainly in faeces and partly in urine. Common side effects are visual disturbances and headache. Avoidance of exposure to light is essential up to 5 days after the therapy.

Tissue Type Plasminogen Activator (tPA)

It is a current concept in the management of ARMD with submacular haemorrhage. Approximately, 10 microgram tPA in 0.1 ml solution is introduced through the retinotomy hole (close to macula) and is kept in contact with clot for 45 minutes. A small quantity of perfluorocarbon liquid is placed on the retinotomy site to keep the tPA in deep contact with the clot. After 45 minutes, the perfluorocarbon along with liquefied blood is rolled out through retinotomy wound. Finally, the retinotomy wound is closed with endolaser. As regards visual prognosis, it is too early to comment on the role of this methodology as adequate quantity of data is not yet available.

Viscoelastic Substances

These are very important substances used during intraocular surgeries. They include methyl cellulose 2%, hydroxy propylmethyl cellulose, chondroitin sulphate and sodium hyaluronate (1%). Sodium hyaluronate is perhaps best, but due to its high cost methyl cellulose is widely used, which is cheaper. These substances are tissue protective, non-toxic, non-antigenic and have molecular weights between thirty thousand and four million Daltons.

They protect corneal endothelium cells from injury during surgical procedures. They artificially maintain the depth of anterior chamber during surgery and also help in performing perfect circular capsulorrhexis.

Therapeutic use: They are used in various surgical procedures like PC IOL, trabeculectomy, full thickness graft, vitreo retinal surgery, etc.

Complications: The most important complication is secondary glaucoma, if it is not properly removed from the operating field after completion of surgery.

Vitreous Substitutes

Common agents used as vitreous substitute are intra-ocular gases, silicon oil and a few miscellaneous substances like sodium hyaluronate, perfluorocarbon liquids, balanced salt solution, etc.

These are used mainly in retinal detachment and vitreous surgery. Commonly used gases are air, xenon, sulfur hexafluoride (SF_6) (Fig.19.5), perfluoropropane (C_3F_8) (Fig. 19.6), perfluoroethane (C_3F_6), etc. These gases expand when placed in eyes and they take longer time to absorb (compared to air). So, they are used to provide a longer lasting tamponade in cases of retinal tears. They are also used in preventive retinopexy for retinal breaks. In extensive detachment of retina, either non-expanding mixture of 86% air + 14% C_3F_8, or 82% air + 18% SF_6 is used.

Complications: Raised IOP, lental change, change in corneal endothelium, entry of gas in subretinal space, etc.

Precautions: Patients with gas in the eyes are advised not to travel by air as high altitude and low atmospheric pressure may cause expansion of gas leading to elevation of IOP. N_2O, if used in general anaesthesia, must be stopped 15-20 minutes prior to administration of intraocular gas.

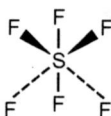

Fig. 19.5. Chemical structure of sulfur hexafluoride

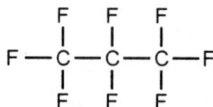

Fig. 19.6. Chemical structure of perfluoropropane

Silicon Oils

Silicon oils (Fig. 19.7) are used in vitreo retinal surgery. But they are very toxic substances and may give rise to raised intraocular tension, cataract, retinopathy, band shaped keratopathy, etc.

$(CH_3)_3 SiO [(C_6H_5) (CH_3) SiO]_n Si (CH_3)_3$

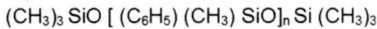

Fig. 19.7. Chemical structure of high-tech silicon oils

The commonest silicon oil used in ophthalmology is a polymer of dimethyl siloxane. Its main use is based on its stable tamponade of retina, particularly after extensive vitrectomy and in the management of giant retinal tears. The tamponade is more effective in upper half of eye ball as it is lighter than water.

Removal: For removal of oil from the globe heavy suction is required.

Perfluorocarbons

Perfluorocarbons like perfluorooctane, perfluorodecalin, perfluorooctylbromide, perfluoroperhydrophenanthrene, etc., are liquids used extensively in retinal detachment surgery. Their main advantage over silicon oil is that they are heavier than water. But these agents are quite retinotoxic and should be removed as completely and quickly as possible.

Various Enzymes Used in Ophthalmology

Hyaluronidase

It is an enzyme which temporarily depolymerizes the mucopolysaccharide, hyaluronic acid (found in interstitial tissue space). It is used along with local anaesthetic lignocaine, details of which have already been discussed.

Alpha Chymotrypsin

This enzyme was once very popular for carrying out enzymic zonulolysis in intra-capsular cataract extraction. It is an obsolete drug today.

Collagenase

It is an enzyme used for debridement of necrotic tissues over burnt areas of skin (precaution is taken not to allow the drug to enter inside the eyes). Usually, a topical antibiotic is used simultaneously. Anticollagenase compounds like sodium EDTA were very popular during early seventies in the management of alkali burn of cornea.

Fibrinolysin Deoxyribonuclease

This combination (fibrnolysin + deoxyribonuclease) attacks fibrin clots and hydrolyses DNA and is very effective as a local debriding agent in cases of burns (care is taken to prevent its entry inside eyes).

Trypsin-chymotrypsin

These enzymes promote earlier recovery in cases of inflammatory edema induced by trauma or any other cause. These enzymes are administered in such a way (enteric coated form) that they survive destructive effect of acid pepsin in stomach and are released in the small intestine from where they are absorbed. After absorption, they bring down the rising plasmin inhibitor levels and help the plasmin to clear up the fibrin blocked microcirculation and gradually the edema disappears and healing starts at an early stage. They are administered half an hour before meals, 1 to 2 lac Armour units (AU) 4 times a day.

Serratiopeptidase

This is another anti-inflammatory enzyme which inhibits the plasmin inhibitors in the same way as trypsin-chymotrypsin. In addition, it destroys histamine, bradykinin and serotonin and so the dilated blood capillaries with permeability defect come back quickly to their normal position. The usual dose is 5 to 10 mg TDPC to be swallowed without crushing by teeth.

Streptokinase and **Urokinase** have already been discussed.

Tissue Glues Used in Ophthalmology

Butyl-2-cyanoacrylate

The most commonly used tissue glue is butyl-2-cyanoacrylate. The moment it comes in contact with tissue fluid, it hardens immediately and so it is useful to seal small corneal perforations. Care is to be taken not to glue other structures like crystalline lens, etc., at the side of perforation. However, it is a temporary emergency measure and wounds larger than 2 to 3 mm are not selected for gluing. Later on, the area affected has to be repaired by a suitable graft.

Fibrin Tissue Adhesive

Another glue used in ophthalmology is fibrin tissue adhesive. This is used to seal corneal perforations, to secure conjunctival and scleral flaps and to repair the traumatic gap created in lens capsule. It is applied with the help of a double barreled syringe, one barrel containing fibrinogen and factor twelve, and the other containing thrombin and calcium. The moment the two fluids come in contact, fibrinogen is converted to fibrin. But the problem with this procedure is that the ingredients must be kept in frozen condition.

Pharmacological Aspects Concerned with Preservation of Cornea

Two popular media for "intermediate term storage" of donor cornea are Optisol and Procell media (storage time: 14 days; temperature: 4°C). The basic ingredients of cornea storage media are dextran 1% (to keep the cornea thin) and chondroitin sulfate (works like glycosaminoglycans of normal cornea). Hepes buffer, electrolytes (simulating aqueous humour composition) and antibiotics (usually gentamicin in 65.5-99 mg/ml concentration) are used. Sometimes vancomycin is also added and some miscellaneous ingredients like insulin, epidermal growth factor, vitamins (particularly Vit. C and Vit. B$_{12}$), antioxidants (e.g. purpuroguallin), anticollagenases, antiproteases, amino acids and hydrocortisone in low concentration are used.

For long term storage, organ culture methodology (can preserve the cornea up to 35 days) and cryopreservation technology (can preserve for indefinite period) are utilized. But at present, cryopreservation is not a desirable technique as there is appreciable endothelial cell loss in spite of using cryoprotective agents like dimethyl sulfoxide (DMSO), glycerol, polivinylpyrolidine, etc.

Antimigraine Drugs

Pharmacotherapy of Migraine

Cases of migraine attending eye clinics can be divided into 3 groups – mild cases, moderate cases and severe cases.

Mild cases usually get less than one attacks per month, which is not unbearable and lasts for about 8 hours. Moderate cases usually get more than one attack, which is unbearable, associated with nausea and vomiting and lasts for 6 to 24 hours. Severe cases usually get more than 2 to 3 attacks per month, which are incapacitating, associated with vertigo, nausea and vomiting lasts for about 12-48 hours.

For mild cases usually a prostaglandin synthesis inhibitor along with an antiemetic is sufficient. For moderate cases, a combination of PG synthesis inhibitors is sufficient. However, some cases may need either an ergot preparation or sumatriptan along with an antiemetic. Severe cases usually respond to an ergot alkaloid or sumatriptan along with an antiemetic.

Prophylactic Therapy of Migraine

Usual drugs used for prophylaxis of migraine are beta adrenergic blockers, calcium channel blockers and tricyclic antidepressants.

Some Common Antimigraine Drugs

Newer drugs of migraine therapy are zolmitriptan, rizatriptan, naratriptan, etc. Drugs under trial are frovatriptan, almotriptan, eletriptan, etc.

Ergot alkaloids

Ergotamine and dihydroergotamine are the most effective ergot alkaloids used in the management of migraine. Both act in the same way. They act by stimulating 5-HT!D/!B receptors in and around the dilated cranial vessels and constrict them thus aborting the attack. They also reduce the neurogenic inflammation. Caffeine (100 mg) helps in the absorption of ergot alkaloids. Ergotamine is usually given orally 1 mg at half hourly intervals till headache subsides, but never exceeding a dose of 6 mg. The most important side effect is vomiting. Ergot alkaloids have no prophylactic role and chronic use of these drugs is risky. The important problems are development of thrombosis and gangrene.

Sumatriptan

Sumatriptan (Fig. 19.8) is a currently used drug. It is better tolerated than ergotamine. It suppresses the vomiting effect of migraine unlike ergot alkaloids (which stimulate the vomiting effect). Headache usually subsides within 2 to 3 hours. Sumatriptan and ergotamine should never be used together. There should be a gap of at least 24 hours between their administration. Sumatriptan selectively stimulates 5HT1D/1B receptor of the dilated cranial vessels and constricts them. It also suppresses the neurogenic inflammation of cranial vessels. Usual oral dose is 50 to 100 mg, which may be repeated after 24 hours. Common side effects are weakness, paraesthesia of extremities, dizziness, etc. The most serious side effect is coronary constriction leading to myocardial infarction.

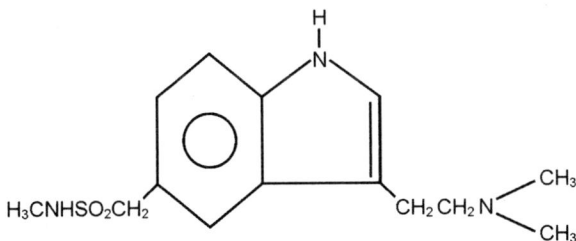

Fig. 19.8. Chemical structure of sumatriptan

Drugs Used for Migraine Prophylaxis

Flunarizine

It is believed to be a cerebroselective calcium channel blocker and possibly blocks the entry of excess calcium in brain cells which protects them from ill effects of hypoxia. The usual oral dose is 10-20 mg once daily.

Propranolol

It is the most commonly used drug. Mechanism of migraine prophylaxis is not yet understood. The initial dose is 40 mg BD which can be gradually increased to 160 mg BD. The antimigraine effect is appreciated within 4 weeks.

Amitriptyline

It is a tricyclic antidepressant. But the mechanism of migraine prophylaxis is not well understood. The usual oral dose is 25 to 50 mg at bed time. This drug suits best the patients suffering from mental depression.

CHAPTER 20

Immunosuppressives and Immunostimulants

Immunosuppressive Agents

Immunosuppressive agents are used to suppress both cell-mediated and humoral immune responses in various ocular immunological diseases and corneal grafting surgery.

Classification

Immunosuppressive agents may be divided into the following classes:
1. *Corticosteroids*
2. *Antineoplastic drugs*: (a) Azathioprine, (b) Methotrexate, (c) Cyclophosphamide, (d) Chlorambucil and (e) Mycophenolate mofetil (MMF)
3. *Inhibitors of T lymphocytes*: a) Cyclosporin, (b) Tacrolimus, (c) Rapamycin and (d) Some newer antibiotics like brequiner, mizoribine, etc.
4. *Miscellaneous agents*: a) Sulfones, (b) Antilymphocytic serum (ALS), (c) Monoclonal antibodies, (d) Leflunomide, (e) Bromocriptine, (f) Colchicine and (g) Daclizumab

Mechanism of Immunosuppressive Action of Some Important Agents

Corticosteroids
- Less production of IL-2 by T cells; thus proliferation of activated T cell clones is hampered.

- Less production of IL-1 by macrophages; thus suppression of induction phase of immune response.
- Suppression of expression of genes which encode cytokines like IL-1, IL-2, IL-6, TNF alfa, etc.

Azathioprine

Azathioprine (Fig. 20.1) is a purine antimetabolite and acts as a powerful immunosuppressive agent by:

- damaging DNA of immunological cells
- selective antagonisation of T lymphocytes
- suppression of cytolytic lymphocytes

The overall primary response is suppression of cell-mediated immunity.

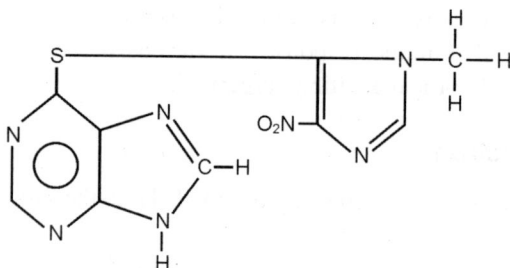

Fig. 20.1. Chemical structure of azathioprine

Methotrexate

It is a folate antagonist and as an immunosuppressant it has three basic functions:

(i) Suppression of cytokine production.

(ii) Suppression of cellular immunity.

(iii) Powerful anti-inflammatory action.

Cyclophosphamide

Cyclophosphamide (Fig. 20.2) is a nitrogen mustard group of drug. As an immunosuppressive agent it suppresses humoral immunity (B cell) more than cell-mediated immunity (T cell)

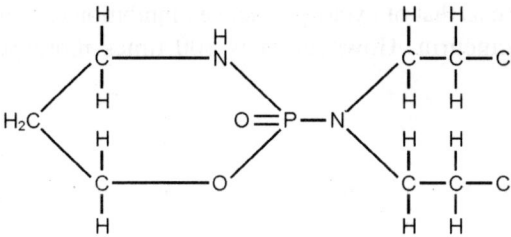

Fig. 20.2. Chemical structure of cyclophosphamide

Chlorambucil

It is a slow acting alkylating agent and is particularly effective on lymphoid tissue. As an immunosuppressive agent, it is a relatively weak agent.

Mycophenolate mofetil (MMF)

It is a prodrug of mycophenolic acid which specifically depresses the synthesis of guanosine nucleotides in both T and B lymphocytes by suppressing the enzyme inosine monophosphate dehydrogenase. In this way, it acts as an immunosuppressive agent.

Cyclosporin

It is an immunosuppressive antibiotic. The possible mechanism of action is:

- It specific inhibits proliferation of T lymphocytes and they are arrested in G_0 or G_1 phase.
- It inhibits response of inducer T cells to IL-1.
- At cellular level, cyclosporin binds to a specialized protein called cyclophilin, and the complex thus formed inactivates a compound called calcineurin inside the target cell. Due to this phenomenon, helper T cells fail to respond to any antigenic stimulus. But suppressor T cells are usually unaffected.

Tacrolimus

It is a new chemical compound structurally different from cyclosporine, but as an immunosuppressive agent its mechanism of action is same as that of cyclosporine, i.e., inhibition of helper T cells through calcineurin. However, it is 100 times more potent than cyclosporin.

Rapamycin

It is a popular macrolide antibiotic which causes immunosuppression by:
- Inhibition of amplification of T cell.
- Obstruction of responses of T cells to IL-2 & IL-4
- Suppression of macrophage activation.

Sulfones

Mechanism of immunosuppressive action in this case involves:
- Inhibition of release of lysosomal enzyme from granulocytes.
- Effect of sulfones on the alternative complement chain.

Antilymphocytic serum

It is prepared from horse's serum immunized by human lymphocytes or fetal thymic tissue. Mechanism of action involves combination of ALS to a specific protein on T lymphocytes surface resulting in a violent antigen-antibody reaction and activation of complement system. The whole phenomenon ultimately leads to lysis of cells (T lymphocytes).

Monoclonal antibodies

Muromonab CD3 is a murine monoclonal antibody which obstructs the participation of T lymphocytes in immunological responses. Ultimately, T lymphocytes disappear from circulation.

Leflunomide

It suppresses the T lymphocytic response to IL-2.

Bromocriptine

It is a potent dopamine antagonist and reduces prolactin release from pituitary. Prolactin modifies immune responses via T lymphocytes. This is the basic mechanism of immunosuppressive action of bromocriptine.

Colchicine

This particular alkaloid gets bound to fibrillar protein tubulin and suppresses granulocytic migration and inhibits release of a specialized glycoprotein. This property has been utilized for immunosuppression in some immunological eye diseases.

Daclizumab

It is a monoclonal human antibody, prepared by genetical engineering of human IgG. It specifically binds to alpha chain of IL-2 receptors. It is a recently introduced immunosuppressive agent.

Immunosuppressive Therapy in Ocular Conditions

1. Uveitis group

(a) *Severe uveitis of unknown origin not responding to usual treatment*: Cyclosporin and methotrexate are commonly used.

(b) *Recurring anterior uveitis*: The commonly used immuno-suppressives are azathioprine, cyclophosphamide, methotrexate, chlorambucil, etc.

(c) *Chronic cyclitis*: Immunosuppressives used are methotrexate, chlorambucil, etc.

(d) *Obstinate type of pars planitis*: Common immunosuppressives used are cyclosporin, azathioprine.

(e) *Sympathetic ophthalmia*: Common immunosuppressives used along with steroids are cyclosporine, azathioprine, methotrexate, cyclophosphamide, chlorambucil, etc.

(f) *Behcet's disease*: Common drugs used are steroids, cyclophosphamide, cyclosporine, colchicines, chlorambucil, etc.

(g) *Vogt-Koyanagi-Harada syndrome*: Drugs commonly used are steroids, azathioprine, cyclosporine, etc.

2. Conjunctival diseases

(a) Acute vernal keratoconjunctivitis not responding to conventional treatment shows improvement with cyclosporine 2% eye drops.

(b) Cicatricial ocular pemphigoid lesions respond to steroids, azathioprine, dapsone, cyclophosphamide, etc.

3. Corneal conditions

(a) *Keratoplasty*: Details have already been discussed.

(b) *Mooren's ulcer*: Common drugs used are cyclosporine, cycloposphamide, etc.

(c) *Connective tissue diseases induced peripheral ulcerative keratitis*: The drug of choice is cyclophosphamide.

4. Scleral diseases

Severe acute scleritis not getting controlled with steroid therapy alone responds well to methotrexate.

5. Miscellaneous conditions involving eye

(a) *Myasthenia gravis*: Drugs used are steroids, azathioprine, cyclosporine, etc.

(b) *Thyroid ophthalmopathy*: Drugs used are steroids, cyclosporin, azathioprine, etc.

(c) *Pseudotumour orbit*: Common drugs used are steroids and methotrexate.

(d) *Idiopathic sclerosing orbital inflammation*: Drugs used are systemic steroids with cyclosporin or azathioprine.

(e) *Tolosa-Hunt syndrome*: Steroids and cyclophosphamide are usually used.

Side effects

Local ocular side effects are superficial punctate keratopathy, chemical conjunctivitis, blockage of punctum and canaliculi, cataract formation, and damage to retina and optic nerve.

Systemic side effects of various cytotoxic agents taken together include bone marrow depression, mutation of genes, chance of neoplastic diseases like lymphomas and lukemias (particularly noted with alkylating agents), teratogenic effect, secondary saprophytic infection, testicular dysfunction (particularly seen with cyclophosphamide and chlorambucil), ulcerative enterocolitis (particularly seen with metabolic antagonists and colchicines), haemorrhagic cystitis (commonly seen with cyclophosphamide), loss of hair (common with cyclophosphamide and methotrexate), hepatic dysfunction (seen particularly with azathioprine, methotrexate and chlorambucil), cardiomyopathy (mainly seen with daunorubicin and doxorubicin), interstitial pulmonary fibrosis (particularly associated with cyclophosphamide, methotrexate), etc.

Amongst other immunosuppressives, cyclosporine is nephrotoxic, ALS may produce hypersensitive reactions and lymphomas, sulfones are hepatotoxic and may cause haemolytic anaemia, leucopenia, etc. Side effects of corticosteroids have already been discussed in a previous chapter.

Doses of Some Important Immunosuppressives Used for Ophthalmic Purpose

- Azathioprine – 1 to 2.5 mg per kg per day orally.
- Methotrexate – 5 to 15 mg per week orally, I.M. or I.V.
- Cyclophosphamide – 1 to 2 mg per kg per day orally, I.V. A pulse therapy I.V. – 750 mg per m^2 is also used sometimes.
- Chlorambucil – 0.1 to 0.2 mg per kg body weight per day orally, but never exceeding a dose of 12-18 mg per day.
- Tacrolimus – 0.1 to 0.15 mg per kg body weight per day orally.
- Cyclosporine – 5 to 7 mg per kg body weight per day orally to start with followed by 1-4 mg per kg body weight per day orally as maintenance dose.
- Antilymphocytic serum (ALS) – 20 to 40 mg per kg body weight per day I.V. for a period of 1 to 2 weeks.
- Dapsone – 25 to 50 mg BD or TD orally.
- Colchicine – The dose should not exceed 0.5 to 0.6 mg BD orally.
- Procarbazine – 50 to 100 mg per day orally.

Post-operative Immunosuppressive Therapy in Penetrating Keratoplasty

After carefully observing the IOP:

(a) Rimexolone 1% ophthalmic suspension is started 6 times a day gradually tailing off to twice per day and then switched over to fluorometholone acetate 0.1% eye drop once daily for a prolonged period depending on clinical condition. No systemic steroid should be used.

(b) Ciprofloxacin 0.3% eye drop is used if there is any epithelial defect.

(c) In poor cases, where there is a chance of graft rejection, cyclosporin is started topically 2% along with systemically 3 to 6 mg per kg body weight. After 4 weeks, the dose of cyclosporin is gradually tailed off to 2 mg per kg body weight which can be continued for 6 months.

Precautions during immunosuppressive therapy

Periodic check up of blood is mandatory. Initially, it is done at intervals of two weeks and later at 4 weeks interval. It should be ensured that:

(a) Total WBC count does not fall below 3500/mm^3.

(b) Polymorph count does not fall below 1500/mm^3.

(c) Platelet count does not go below 75,000/mm^3.

Recent Advances in Immunosuppressive Therapy

Recently, two new immunosuppressives have been approved for use in the USA:

(a) Inflixmab—It is an anti TNFα-monoclonal antibody and is allowed for use in cases of rheumatiod arthritis (along with methotrexate), and in resistant cases (not responding to conventional treatment) of Crohn's disease.

(b) Etanercept—Although it is not a monoclonal antibody, it resembles infliximab in its function. It has been permitted for use in cases of rheumatoid arthritis (along with methotrexate).

Both these drugs are highly toxic and may produce serious infections of upper respiratory tract and urinary tract.

As all immunosuppressive drugs have side effects, a new concept of immunological tolerance to a specific antigen (e.g. in case of a transplant) is coming up. The developments are in the experimental stages (in animal models mainly) and so only the broad approaches are indicated below:

(a) Soluble HLA thrapy

(b) Specific antigen in peptide form therapy

(c) Restriction of co-stimulating signal

(d) A totally new type of reconstruction of the immune system prior to transplantation (mainly bone marrow or stem cell)

Immunostimulants

These agents are used to increase immunity against various infections like AIDS, herpes, mycotic infections, toxoplasmosis and certain malignant conditions like melanoma.

Use of Immunostimulants in Ophthalmology

Immunostimulants have been found to be useful in ophthalmology in a number of situations. Some of the uses are listed below:

(a) Use of ampligen which has a chemical structure of mismatched double stranded RNA, in CMV and HIV infections. It stimulates production of endogenous lymphokines.

(b) Use of interleukin-2 (IL-2) in AIDS and melanoma. It stimulates proliferation of activated T lymphocytes and maturation of natural and lymphokinin activated killer cells.

(c) Inosine pranobex has been found to be effective against herpes simplex, herpes zoster and cytomegalo virus infections by stimulating both T and B lymphocytes.

(d) Thymic factor isolated from thymus enhances T lymphocytic functions and is used in many viral infections and immunodeficiency states.

(e) Interferon alpha can stimulate T lymphocytes, NK-cells and macrophages and has been found to be useful in many viral infections and Kaposi's sarcoma.

(f) BCG vaccination is found to stimulate T cells and NK-cells and has been found to be useful against many malignant conditions like melanoma.

(g) Resistant cases of atopic keratoconjunctivitis respond well to I.V. immune-globulin therapy.

(h) Viral infections like cytomegalovirus and herpes zoster can be treated by transfer factor obtained from activated lymphocytes.

(i) Small doses of retinal and uveal antigen therapy can make an individual immunotolerant against these agents and this principle has been found to be effective against chronic relapsing uveitis.

(j) Role of thalidomide and levamisole as immunostimulant is under trial in many ophthalmologic conditions.

CHAPTER 21

Antineoplastics and Radiotherapy in Ophthalmology

Antineoplastic Drugs

Therapeutics of malignancy is still in its infancy. However, there are some drugs which suppress the replication or maturation of rapidly proliferating neoplastic cells. But at the same time some host cells (viz. blood cells, immunological cells, etc.) are also affected.

Chemical Classification

These can be classified as follows:

1. *Alkylating agents*: These agents form covalent bonds with DNA and thus they hamper the transcription and replication phenomenon of rapidly dividing cells. They are divided into following subgroups:

  (a) Nitrogen mustards, e.g., Cyclophosphamide, Chlorambucil, Melphalan.
  (b) Ethylenimine, e.g., Thio-tepa & Methylmelamines, e.g., hexamethylmelamine.
  (c) Nitrosoureas, e.g., Carmustine, Streptozocine, etc.
  (d) Alkyl Sulfonates, e.g., Busulfan, etc.
  (e) Triazenes, e.g., dacarbazine.

2. *Antimetabolites*: They interfere with the metabolic pathway involved in synthesis of nucleic acids.

  They are divided into following subgroups:

  (a) Folic acid antagonists, e.g., methotrexate.
  (b) Purine antagonists, e.g., 6-mercaptopurine, thioguanine, etc.
  (c) Pyrimidine antagonists, e.g., cytosine arabinoside, 5-fluorouracil (Fig. 21.1).

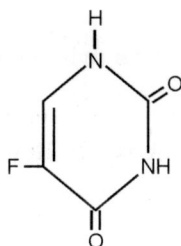

Fig. 21.1. Chemical structure of 5-fluorouracil

3. *Vinca alkaloids*: These alkaloids (e.g. vinblastine) are of plant origin and they interfere with the formation of mitotic spindle by inhibiting the microtubule function.
4. *Antibiotics*: These antibiotics prevent eukaryotic cell division, e.g., bleomycin, mitomycin C, dactinomycin, etc.
5. *Enzymes*, e.g., L-asparaginase: The amino acid L-asparagine is not essential in extra amounts for multiplication of normal cells, as adequate amount is synthesized in the body itself. But for rapidly proliferating cells extra amount has to be synthesized. The enzyme L-asparaginase can block the synthesis of L-asparagine in the tumour cells and so their growth and multiplication is retarded.
6. *Hormones and hormone antagonists*: Hormones used in different types of neoplastic conditions are glucocorticoids, androgens, oestrogen, etc. Hormone antagonists include tamoxifen, flutamide, etc.
7. *Heavy metal derivatives*: e.g., Cisplatin (Fig. 21.2).
8. *Radioactive isotopes:* e.g., radioactive iodine (^{131}I), radioactive gold (^{198}Au), radioactive phosphorus (^{32}P), etc.

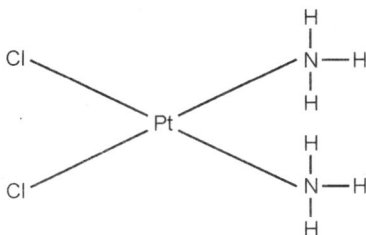

Fig. 21.2. Chemical structure of cisplatin

9. *Miscellaneous agents:* e.g., hydroxyurea, interferon, monoclonal antibodies and special radioactive isotopes (^{125}Iodine), ^{192}Iridium , ^{60}Cobalt , ^{106}Ruthenium, etc.)

Uses of Antineoplastic Drugs in Ophthalmology

- 5-Fluorouracil ointment (5%) has been used in the management of skin lesions around eyes like hyperkeratosis, squamous cell carcinoma, basal cell carcinoma, etc.
- Various cytotoxic agents are used in the management of malignant tumours (usually in association with radiotherapy) like retinoblastoma, malignant melanoma (occasionally), lymphomas, rhabdomyosarcoma, neuroblastoma, etc.
- Both 5-fluorouracil (5-FU) and mitomycin C are used intraoperatively during glaucoma surgery to prevent scarring of filtering bleb. The concentration of 5-FU used is 50 mg per ml and that of mitomycin C is 0.2 to 0.5 mg per ml. Although mitomycin C is preferred by surgeons, it is more toxic than 5-FU. Many cases of avascular blebs with complications like extreme hypotony, wound leak, macular edema and endophthalmitis are found to occur when mitomycin C is used.
- 5-FU in a dose of 0.5 mg injected into vitreous cavity has been used in the prophylaxis and treatment of vitreoretinal proliferations. Other drugs used for this purpose include corticosteroids, daunorubicin, fluorouridine, colchicines, etc.
- Mitomycin C (0.02-0.04%) and thiotepa (0.05%) are used locally in the prophylaxis of recurrence of pterygium after its surgical removal.
- Many cytotoxic agents are used for immunosuppression.

Ocular side effects

These may be conjunctival irritation, punctate keratopathy, blockage of nasolacrimal passage, uveitis, cataract, retinopathy, maculopathy, optic neuritis, etc.

Contraindications

Important contraindications are pregnancy, acute illness (like tuberculosis, severe fungal infection, etc.), peptic ulceration, etc.

Retinoblastoma

Standard Regime of Drugs Used for Chemotherapy of Retinoblastoma

The important drugs used nowadays are:
- Vincristine – 0.05 mg/kg
- Carboplatin – 18 mg/kg
- Teniposide – 7.7 mg/kg
- Etoposide – 3-5 mg/kg

The present day concept is to use at least 3 drugs at a time for 3-14 days. Thereafter, the therapy is again repeated after sometime and several such cycles the required.

Radiotherapy and Retinoblastoma

It is a highly radiosensitive tumour and following techniques are usually used:

(a) *External beam radiotherapy (EBRT)*: Radiation used is 3500 to 4500 rads, spread over a period of 5 weeks approximately. It is not practiced nowadays due to complications resulting from radiation of whole eye.

(b) *Plaque radiotherapy (PR)*: It is widely practiced. The duration of treatment is usually 2½ days. Radioactive isotopes like [125]Iodine, [192]Iridium, [60]Cobalt, [106]Ruthenium, etc., are used for this purpose. Out of these, [125]Iodine is most popular.

Drugs used for chemotherapy of uveal malignant melanoma

The main drugs used are dacarbazine, vincristine, thiotepa, cisplatin, interferon alpha, etc. A new method of treatment called photodynamic therapy has been introduced recently where photosensitizers like benzoporphyrin are used.

Plaque radiotherapy for malignant uveal melanoma

The isotopes used are [60]Cobalt, [109]Ruthenium, [198]Gold, [125]Iodine, [192]Iridium, etc.

Drugs used for chemotherapy of conjunctival malignant melanoma after surgical removal

(a)   *Topical chemotherapy*: Commonly used drug is mitomycin C-0.04%, 4 times a day × 28 days to prevent recurrences.

(b)   *Generalized chemotherapy*: Drug combination used is either lomustine plus bleomycin plus vincristine, or dacarbazine alone or in combination with tamoxifen.

Drugs used for chemotherapy of malignant melanoma of lids

After surgical resection, chemotherapy is usually done with carboplatin, daarbazine, lomustine, etc. Concurrent radiotherapy plus interferon alpha therapy is more effective.

Drugs used to treat squamous cell carcinoma of conjunctiva

After surgical removal of the mass, topical 5-fluorouracil 1% eye drop (1 drop 4 times a day x 3 weeks) shows good results.

Drugs used to treat basal cell carcinoma

Cisplatin I.V. can reduce the bulk of tumour and then the tumour can be excised followed by radiotherapy. Finally, a combination course of cisplatin and doxorubicin is used.

CHAPTER 22

Chelating Agents

The agents which form non-toxic complexes with toxic metals and inhibit the binding of metallic cations with body ligands and help in their excretion are called chelating agents.

Important chelating agents used in ophthalmology are:

- Dimercaprol (British Anti Lewisite; BAL) and succimer.
- d-Penicillamine, acetyl d-penicillamine, Trientine.
- Desferrioxamine and Deferiprone.
- Calcium disodium edetate.

Dimercaprol

Dimercaprol (Fig. 22.1) is mainly effective against metals which attack sulfhydryl containing enzyme system, e.g., As, Hg, Cu, Au, etc.

Preparations and dose: Dimercaprol injection 100 mg/2 ml (in arachis oil). In arsenic and mercury poisoning, it is given I.M., 5 mg/kg as a loading dose followed by 2-3 mg/kg at intervals of 4 to 8 hours for next 2 days. Thereafter, the same amount is repeated as maintenance dose, once a day × 10 days. Urine is made alkaline to facilitate the excretion of metal chelate.

In copper poisoning, it is used as an adjuvant to d-penicillamine in the dosage 300 mg/day I.M. injection × 10 days at 2 months intervals.

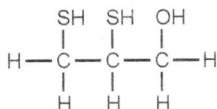

$$\underset{\underset{H}{|}}{\overset{\overset{SH}{|}}{C}} - \underset{\underset{H}{|}}{\overset{\overset{SH}{|}}{C}} - \underset{\underset{H}{|}}{\overset{\overset{OH}{|}}{C}}$$

Fig. 22.1. Chemical structure of dimercaprol

Side effects: Side effects are mild like G.I. tract irritation, rise in B.P., rise in heart rate, headache, burning sensation all over the body, etc. The side effects can be counteracted to a large extent by administration of antihistaminics (H1 blocker), 30 minutes prior to administration of dimercaprol.

Succimer

It is similar to dimercaprol chemically, but is orally effective. It is used mainly in lead poisoning and its side effects are also less than those of dimercaprol.

d-Penicillamine

d-Penicillamine (Fig. 22.2) can chelate Cu, Pb, Hg, etc. A derivative of d-penicillamine, called acetyl d-penicillamine is used to treat Hg poisoning mainly. Patients who are allergic to d-Penicillamine can be treated by a newly introduced compound trientine.

Preparations and dose: Cap. d-penicillamine (150 mg and 250 mg).

The usual dose in Wilson's disease is 1 to 2 g daily in divided doses, orally half an hour before meals. Thereafter, the maintenance dose is 0.75 to 1g/day depending on response.

Side effects: Important side effects are hypersensitive reactions, pemphigoid lesions, bone marrow depression, and pyridoxine deficiency (and so pyridoxine 25 mg per day is prescribed along with d-penicillamine).

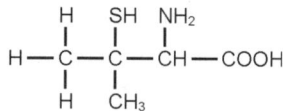

$$
\begin{array}{ccc}
H & SH & NH_2 \\
| & | & | \\
H - C - C - CH - COOH \\
| & | \\
H & CH_3
\end{array}
$$

Fig. 22.2. Chemical structure of d-penicillamine

Desferrioxamine

Desferrioxamine (Fig. 22.3) is a popular iron chelater obtained from Stremtomyces pilosus. 1g can chelate 85 mg of elemental iron. It is administered parenterally.

Preparations with dose: Inj. Desferrioxamine 500 mg vial. In transfusion siderosis (as found in thalassemia due to excessive blood

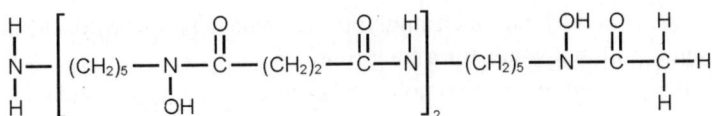

Fig. 22.3. Chemical structure of desferrioxamine

transfusion), the usual dose is 0.5 to 1g/day I.M. It may also be given I.V. along with the transfused blood.

In siderosis bulbi 10% solution by sub conjunctival injection (0.5 ml. – twice per week × 3 to 10 weeks) has been tried with encouraging results.

Side effects: Important side effects are anaphylactic shock, renal damage, hepatic damage and neurotoxicities.

A recently introduced iron chelating agent is Deferiprone, which is orally effective and cheap. But it is not as powerful as desferrioxamine.

Calcium Disodium Edetate (CaNa₂EDTA)

The basic pharmacological action of this compound is chelation, mobilization and removal of metals like Pb, Cu, Zn, and some radioactive metals, but beneficial action is seen in Pb poisoning. It is administered parenterally.

The usual dose in Pb poisoning is 1g dissolved in 200 to 300 ml of 5% dextrose, to be infused for more than one hour twice per day × 3 to 5 days. A second course may be needed after 5 to 7 days. The most dangerous side effect is renal proximal tubular necrosis.

Important Uses of Chelating Agents in Ophthalmology

1. *Siderosis bulbi*: This is seen in cases where an iron foreign body is lodged inside the eye which could not be removed. There is electrolytic dissociation of iron inside the eye which combines with the cells and ultimately destroys them.
2. *Kayser-Fleischer ring*: Associated with Wilson's disease or chalcosis.
3. *Mercurialentis*: Deposition of Hg on outer lens capsules is found in workers exposed to mercury vapour.

4. Arsenic amblyopia: Such amblyopia is found in people who consume arsenic polluted water for a long time.

5. Lead poisoning: Ophthalmological problems of lead poisoning faced by workers of various industries like glass polishers, enamel workers, lead paint manufacturing industries, plumbers, etc. The important ocular features are optic neuritis, retinopathy, internal ophthalmoplegia, etc.

CHAPTER 23

Vitamins and Antioxidants

Vitamins are substances, usually derived from food sources (some are synthesized in the system also), that form important constituents of various enzyme systems essential for life process to continue. Deficiency usually occurs due to increased demand (e.g. pregnancy, lactation, etc.), decreased supply (due to poverty), interference with absorption (e.g. malabsorption syndrome, prolonged use of liquid, paraffin, etc.) and due to drug interactions (e.g. INH interferes with conversion of pyridoxal to pyridoxal phosphate, folic acid utilization may be hampered by diphenythydantoin, etc.)

Conventionally vitamins are divided into 2 groups: (i) fat soluble (A, D, E, K) and (ii) water soluble (B complex and C). Out of these, vitamin K (from ophthalmologist's point of view) has been already dealt with in earlier chapter (Chapter 19).

Vitamin A

Vitamin A_1, called retinol, is present in liver oils (cod liver, halibut liver), egg yolk, milk, butter, etc. Vitamin A_2, called dehydroretinol, is found in sweet water fishes like rohu, katla, etc. Green leafy vegetables, carrots, spinach, tomato, pumpkin, etc., contain provitamin A, called carotene (the most active being beta-carotene). One molecule of beta-carotene yields two molecules of retinol. But such a high conversion rate does not occur inside the human system and after a prolonged survey most of the pharmacologists have concluded that 1 retinol equivalent means intake of 6 microgram of dietary carotene.

Pharmacokinetic Considerations

The dietary retinol usually remains in the form of an ester – retinyl palmitate. Hydrolysis of the ester occurs in lumen of the intestine (by pancreatic enzymes) and also in the brush borders of intestinal epithelial cells. Then operation of a carrier-mediated process starts, aided by CRBP (cellular retinol binding protein) and retinol gains entry inside the intestinal cells, where esterification to palmitate occurs. Palmitate thus formed is incorporated in chylomicrons and stored in hepatic cells. But poor availability of bile and protein hampers such an absorption process. After the liver is fully saturated, the retinyl esters are once again hydrolyzed and retinol thus formed gets bound to a special alpha-one globulin, called RBP (retinol binding protein), which is prepared by hepatic cells and then retinol RBP complex forms another complex with transthyretin (which is actually a thyroxine binding pre albumin) and the whole complex circulates in the blood to reach its destination, i.e., target sites. After getting attached to cell where a complex with CRBP is formed, this retinol CRBP complex acts as a cellular reservoir which releases retinol wherever there is a demand in the target organs – be it retina or bones or epithelial cells, etc.

In retina it is converted to 11-cis-retinal, which is utilized to form rhodopsin. But in other target organs it is converted to retinoic acid which enters the target cell nucleus and gets attached to two specific receptors RARs and RXRs along with CRABP (cellular retinoic acid binding protein). Finally, a part of retinol is reutilized through enterohepatic circulation and a small part is excreted in urine and faeces.

The normal level of plasma retinol is 30 to 70 microgram per dl. This is maintained for a long time even if the individual is suffering from lack of vitamin A because the hepatic reserve releases the stored retinyl esters (the average amount of such stored retinyl ester in human liver is 100 to 300 microgram/ gram). When all the reserved store is exhausted and the plasma level of retinol comes down below 10 to 20 microgram/dl, night blindness and other associated features of vitamin A deficiency appear in the individual.

Vitamin A and Vision

Retina receives 11-cis-retinol which is converted into 11-cis-retinal helped by pyridine nucleotides in a double way reaction. 11-cis-Retinal thus formed combines with a protein called 'opsin' to form rhodopsin which is mostly stored in the membranes of the disc, present in outer segments of rods.

When a photon of light falls on a rhodopsin molecule, the latter gets bleached with the formation of a series of intermediates ultimately resulting in the formation of all-trans-retinal and detached opsin molecule. Activated rhodopsin combines with a specialized protein present in outer segments of rods, called Transducin (Gt), which is a G protein. This transducin through a series of reactions involving cyclic GMP ultimately sets up a primary receptor potential. And finally, action potentials are generated which transverse to areas 17,18,19 of cerebral cortex via visual pathway.

The all-trans retinal is reutilized. Either it is directly isomerized to 11-cis-retinal or through a cord line converted to all-trans-retinol, then to 11-cis-retinol and finally to 11-cis-retinal. 11-cis-retinal then combines with opsin to regenerate visual purple (rhodopsin). The photochemistry of vision is illustrated in Fig. 23.1.

When plasma level of retinol goes below 20 micrograms/dl, there is fall in level of rhodopsin and retinol in retina, leading to the earliest manifesting symptom – night blindness. Prompt elevation of plasma retinol level leads to quick recovery from the problem, but delay in treatment may lead to degeneration of opsin and subsequent degeneration of outer segments of rods occurs leading to permanent blindness. One should also take care to improve the nutritional status of protein intake as opsin is a protein.

Similar types of sequences of events happen in cones also. The protein portions in cones are different and are called idopsin. Three types of cone pigments have been further specifically identified. These are cyanolabe, chlorolabe and erythrolabe which exhibit maximum sensitivity to wavelengths of 450, 535 and 570 nm, respectively, which roughly correspond to blue, green and red parts of visual spectrum.

Vitamin A and Other Biological Functions

The structural and functional integrities of epithelial cells are maintained by vitamin A. It has an important role in epithelial differentiation, promotion of mucous secretion, prevention of hyperkeratinisation and improved capacity to resist infection. Animal experiments have shown that vitamin A has antitumour activity. A detailed investigation has shown specifically that vitamin A does not have any direct cytotoxic action but can modify the phenotype which may be responsible for producing a malignant lesion.

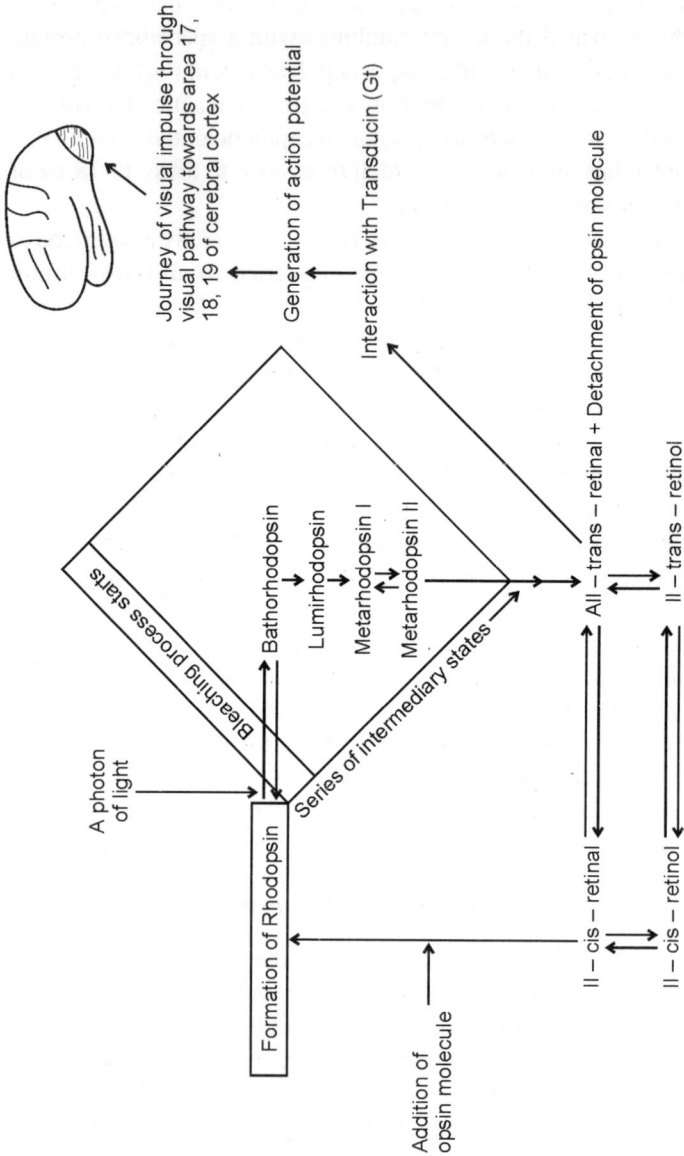

Fig. 23.1. Diagram illustrating photochemistry of vision

Vitamin A can modify the effect of some hormones and growth factors by influencing the expression of receptors. Vitamin A, by influencing the rhythm of action of osteoblasts, can affect bone growth. For example, its deficiency may cause reduction in the size of spinal and cranial foramina (leading to nerve compression syndrome) and its high concentration causes rarefaction and resorption of bone. Experimental models have shown that in the case of CMI (cell-mediated immunity), vitamin A deficiency inhibits both splenic lymphocytic proliferation and capacity of cytotoxic action of killer cells. However, clinically it was found that vitamin A administration to children with measles reduced mortality and morbidity. After this pharmacoepidomiological survey, a joint notice by WHO and UNICEF was issued in 1987 stating that all children with measles should receive (100 thousand to 200 thousand IU of vitamin A (according to age) in countries where fatality rate is 1% or more.

Clinical Features Associated with Vitamin A Deficiency

Eye

The basic changes in the eye are due to keratinising metaplasia. It usually coexists with protein energy malnutrition and may also be associated with conditions like prolonged diarrhoea, measles, malabsorption syndrome, etc. The resultant clinical condition is called xerophthalmia (Table 23.1) which may range from night blindness (occurring in about 2 to 5 lac children per year and is called *nutritional blindness*) to phthisis bulbi. Incidence of xerophthalmia mainly occurs within 4 to 6 years of life, the maximum incidence being within 6 months to 3 years of age.

Treatment part of such conditions will be discussed in the later part of this chapter.

Skin

Hyperkeratinisation, dryness, papular eruptions and atrophy of sweat glands of skin are the basic findings.

Bones

Effects of vitamin A deficiency on bones have already been discussed.

Table 23.1. Classification of clinical features of xerophthalmia (after WHO)

Name of the stage	Clinical features
XN (Night blindness)	Earliest manifestation of Vit. A deficiency.
X1A (Xerox of conjunctiva)	Transformation to stratified squamous from columnar epithelium with keratinization and loss of goblet cells.
X1B (Appearance of Bitots spot)	Triangular or oval foamy spots on temporal side. of limbus in interpalpebral fissure.
X2 (Xerosis of cornea)	Cornea becomes dry and lusturelss.
X3A (Keratomalacia involving less than 1/3rd of corneal surface)	Corneal stroma undergoes permanent destruction. Formation of ulcers which may perforate.
X3B (Keratomalacia involving more than 1/3rd of corneal surface)	Such ulcers usually result in formation of anterior staphyloma.
XS (Formation of xerophthalmic scar)	The ultimate result is formation of nebula, macula, leucoma, adherent leucoma, anterior Staphyloma, phthisis bulbi.
XF (Uyemura's fundus)	Constriced visual field with small white lesions on retina.

Sweat glands

Apart from atrophic changes, keratinising squamous cell metaplasia is also found.

Respiratory system

Keratinisation of epithelium, together with lessened mucous secretion leads to increased susceptibility to respiratory tract infection. Elasticity of lung tissue is also diminished.

Urogenital system

There is shredding of malformed epithelial cells in the urinary tract which acts as nidus for calculi formation. It also plays a role in spermatogenesis, maintenance of pregnancy and prevention of teratogenesis.

Gastrointestinal system

The epithelial cells show degenerative changes and there is reduction in the number of goblet cells but keratinisation never occurs. In pancreatic duct epithelium, there is evidence of metaplasia and all these factors jointly are responsible for diarrhoea which is so common in vitamin A deficiency.

Central nervous system

A few cases of Vit A deficiency are associated with various neurological lesions, increased intra-cranial pressure and hydrocephalus.

Erythropoetic system

Defective erythropoesis has been reported in cases of vitamin A deficiency.

Special senses

Hearing and taste sensation may be affected possibly due to keratinizing effect.

Therapeutic Uses

1. *Management of xerophthalmia*: According to the guidelines suggested by WHO, Vit. A should be given orally in the dose 200,000 I.U. with the earliest manifestation of xerophthalmia. Thereafter, the same dose is repeated after 24 hr orally and finally the same dose is repeated within next 1 to 4 weeks. Half of the above dose is recommended for infants of 6 to 11 months of age (or whose body weight is less than 8 kg) and one fourth of the dose should be given to infants, whose age is less than six months. Intramuscular injection is no more encouraged and is kept reserved for those who suffer from diarrhoea, malabsorption syndrome, vomiting, etc. Under these circumstances, intramuscular injection of 100,000 I.U. may be used. Along with this, the eye involved is treated with antibiotics (topical tobramycin preferably) and atropine eye ointment 1%.

2. *Treatment of various dermatological conditions*: For this purpose various synthetic retinoids are used, which activate nuclear receptors and regulate gene transcription. Important dermatological conditions where retinoids are used are leukoplakia and Darier's disease.

3. *Use as anticancer agent*: Many drugs of retinoid group are under investigation. For example, bexarotene has shown promising results in cutaneous T cell lymphoma (CTCL). All trans-retinoic acid produces remission in acute promyelocytic leukemia, etc.

Hypervitaminosis A

Natural as well as synthetic retinoids may produce acute or chronic toxicity depending on the dose consumed, period of consumption and age of the patient.

Acute toxicity features include vomiting, papilloedema, raised intracranial pressure induced acute headache, neurological features (drowsiness, dizziness, etc.), hepatomegally and the most dangerous effect (usually occurring 24 hours after consumption) is generalized peeling of the skin.

Chronic toxicity features are skin lesions (dry desquamated and erythematous lesions), acute pain and tenderness of bones, fall of hairs, pseudotumour cerebri, hyperostosis, etc. In paediatric patients, bulging of fontanelle due to increased intracranial pressure, vomiting, liver damage (from enlarged liver to cirrhosis of liver), hypercalcaemia, elevated plasma alkaline phosphatase (due to increased osteoblastic activity, etc.)

Pharmacoepidemiological survey has shown that adults taking 10 mg vitamin A/ day × 6 months and infants taking 7.5 to 15 mg of retinol/day x 30 days develop the features of chronic toxicity. Similarly, consumption of more than 500 mg in case of adults, 100 mg in a kid and 30 mg in an infant is sufficient to produce acute toxicity features.

Diagnostic plasma level of retinol (for hypervitaminosis A) is >100 microgram/dl. The risk is more in liver diseases and PEM (protein energy malnutrition) as the plasma concentrations of RBP (retinal binding protein) are very low in such cases. Animal experiments have shown that vitamin E can counteract many adverse effects of hypervitaminosis A. So, nowadays it is customary to use vitamin E along with vitamin A to avoid many ill effects of vitamin A.

Vitamin A has teratogenic property also. According to a survey many of the mothers receiving 7.5 to 12 mg of vitamin A/day during first trimester of pregnancy gave birth to babies with congenital anomaly. Synthetic retinoids are even more dangerous as they are stored in body fat. Such patients should be asked to delay conception up to 2 years or even more than that after stoppage of the drug (the classical example is etretinate). Hypervitaminosis never occurs even after high consumption of beta-carotene, because limited amount of carotene is converted into retinol.

Commonly Used Preparations of Vitamin A and Synthetic Retinoids

- Vitamin A tablet containing 50,000 I.U.
- Vitamin A injection containing 100,000 I.U./ml.
- Vitamin A + D capsule containing 4000 I.U. vitamin A and 400 I.U. vitamin D.
- Vitamin A solution containing 50,000 I.U./ml for oral use.
- Tretinoin (retinoic acid) 0.025-0.05% skin cream.
- Adapalene 0.1% gel to be applied only once at bedtime.

Mass Prophylaxis Programme with Oral Vitamin A (Recommended by WHO)

As such vitamin A supplementation is not essential for people taking a balanced diet. However, a prophylactic schedule according to the guidelines suggested by WHO for developing countries is as follows:

Just after birth, the suggested dose for neonate is 50,000 I.U. orally. Thereafter, 100,000 I.U. to be taken once in 4 to 6 months up to the age of 1 year and 200,000 I.U. once in every 4 to 6 months orally in children above the age of one year.

In case of pregnant and lactating mothers, a daily dose of 5,000 I.U. has been suggested. Mothers just after giving birth to child should receive single dose of 300,000 I.U. orally. Such a prophylaxis programme is called mass prophylaxis programmes.

Daily requirements of vitamin A

- For pregnant and lactating mothers: 3,000 to 3,500 I.U.
- For infants up to 4 years of age: 1000 to 1200 I.U.

- For school going children, adolescents and healthy adults: 2250 I.U.

Vitamin D

The main importance of vitamin D lies in the fact that it can cure rickets. By the term vitamin D, we mean a mixture of substance which can cure rickets. In the skin cholecalciferol (vitamin D_3) is formed from 7-dehydrocholesterol by the action of ultraviolet light. Similarly, calciferol (vitamin D_2) is formed from dietary ergosterol (present in mould, yeast, etc.) by the action of ultraviolet rays.

In case of human beings, both vitamins D_2 and D_3 are equally potent. Previously, it was thought that vitamin D must be supplied from outside but present day concept is that vitamin D_3 can be produced in sufficient amounts inside the system following exposure to ultraviolet light of sun. Conversion of 7-dehydrocholesterol to vitamin D involves three main steps:

(a) First step occurs in skin.

(b) Second step occurs in liver.

(c) Third step occurs in kidney.

That is why, nowadays, vitamin D is regarded as a hormone, as it is synthesized in so many places and acts on specific target cells situated elsewhere.

Deficiency of Vitamin D

From the ophthalmologic point of view, hypovitaminosis D may be associated with zonular cataract. This may be associated with features of rickets in children.

In adults, hypovitaminosis D causes osteomalacia. In advanced cases, osteomalacia may precipitate pathological fractures and severe muscular asthenopia. In osteomalacia there is both loss of calcium from bone and phosphate depletion leading to impaired mineralization of bone. In osteoporosis, similar pathological fractures may be the presenting feature but the basic defect in osteoporosis is reduction in bone mass.

In rickets, the children show delay in general development of the stature associated with severe muscular hypotonia. Other characteristic features are rickety rosary (due to formation of swellings of the rib ostochondral junction); delayed closure of anterior fontanelle; bossing of both the parietal and the frontal bones, various types of bony deformities of chest, spine, pelvis long bones, etc. Sometimes in severe hypovitaminosis D, there may be hypocalceimic tetany and epileptic seizures.

Preparations and Doses of Some Important Vitamin D Group of Drugs

1. *Shark liver oil with vitamin D*: It possesses 1000 I.U. of vitamin D and 6000 I.U. of vitamin A per ml; the usual dose is 0.5 to 1.5 ml per day, given orally.
2. *Cholecalciferol injection (Vit D_3):* It is available as 300,000 I.U. per ml in an oily solvent; single injection is given according to severity of condition, which can be repeated after 4 to 6 weeks.
3. *Cholecalciferol granules*: 1g containing 60,000 I.U. is given at intervals of 3 to 4 weeks and then it can be repeated every 2 to 6 months depending upon the clinical condition. 1 microgram of cholecalciferol is equivalent to 40 I.U. of vit. D.
4. *Calciferol (vit. D_2):* Also called ergocalciferol, it is available in 25,000 and 50,000 I.U. capsules. An injection preparation in oil is also available containing 50,000 I.U. per ml. for I.M. injection.
5. *Calcitriol (1, 2-dihydroxycholecalciferol):* It is available as capsule (0.25 or 0.5 microgram) and injection (1 or 2 microgram per ml); the capsule is prescribed either daily or on alternate days.
6. *Dihydrotachysterol (DHT):* A derivative of vit. D_2 prepared synthetically, it is not dependant on PTH induced renal activation; hence, it is a drug of choice in renal rickets and hypoparathyroidism. The usual dose is 0.25 to 0.5 mg per day.
7. *Alfacalcidol (1-alpha - OH D_3):* It is converted in liver to 1, 25 $(OH)_2D_3$, i.e., Calcitriol. Serum calcium monitoring is essential to prevent hypercalcaemia. The usual dose is 1 to 2 microgram per day. In case of children, if the body weight is less than 20 kg, the dose prescribed is 0.5 microgram per day

Therapeutic Uses of Vitamin D

- In the prevention and management of nutritional rickets and osteomalacia.

- In the management of age-related osteoporosis.
- In the management of various other forms of rickets. Vit. D group of drugs are used to treat vit. D dependant rickets (treated with calcitriol or alfacalcidol), Vit.D resistant rickets (treated with phosphate plus calcitriol or alfacalcidol) and renal rickets (treated with calcitriol or alfacaloidol or dihydrotachysterol).
- In some miscellaneous conditions. Conditions like hypoparathyroidism (treated with calcitriol or dihydrotachysterol or alfacalcidol), renal tubular defects with vit. D resistant rickets, osteomalacia and psoriasis (a non-hypercalcaemic derivative of vit. D called calcipotriol is used) are managed with various types of vitamin D group of drugs.

Hypervitaminosis D

Long term administration of a large dose of Vit. D leads to hypervitaminosis D. It is characterized by hypercalcaemia, hyperphosphatemia, generalized demineralization of bones, hypercalciuria and metastatic calcification. Hypercalcaemia generally causes muscular asthenopia, lethargy, nausea, vomiting, anorexia, marked constipation, depressed renal functions, cardiac arrhythmia, mental confusion, and some cases may even pass into coma. The main management line in such conditions is:

- Urgent stoppage of Vit. D group of drugs.
- Maintenance of fluid balance with low calcium intake.
- Use of drugs like glucocorticoids.

Drug Interactions

Antiepileptics like phenytoin and phenobarpitone can reduce the sensitivity of target organs to the effect of calcitriol. Prolonged intake of some other drugs like liquid paraffin and cholestyramine may hamper the absorption of Vit. D.

Vitamin E (Alpha Tocoferol)

Important sources of vitamin E include wheat germ oil, soya bean oil, rice germ oil, green leaves of spinach and lettuce, egg yolk, etc. Average daily requirement of vitamin E is 10 to 30 mg. One mg is equivalent to 1.5 I.U. of Vit E.

Role of Vitamin E

Vitamin E acts as a natural antioxidant and protects biological membrane from the ill effects of free radicals. These free radicals, which are unpaired electrons, and oxidative free radicals, which are produced during various metabolic reactive processes, may damage cellular DNA. Experimental evidences have shown that vitamin E protects PUFA (polyunsaturated fatty acids) present inside membrane phospholipids and circulating lipoproteins. This concept of antioxidant theory stimulated the clinical scientists to prescribe the drugs like beta-carotene, Vit. C and specifically Vit. E in many conditions like coronary artery disease, diabetic retinopathy, macular degenerations, etc. It is true that Vit. E is a powerful antioxidant and has capacity to save biological membrane.

Therapeutic Uses

(A) Ocular conditions

- Used to prevent retinopathy of prematurity (retrotental fibroplasias) in premature infants who were placed under high concentration of oxygen. The usual dose is 100 mg/kg of the body weight given orally per day.
- Other conditions where Vit. E is tried include ARMD, cataract prophylaxis (along with Vit. C), and in protecting corneal endothelial cells, etc.

(B) Non-ocular conditions

- Vitamin E is used along with vitamin A to promote its absorption and storage, and to minimize the risk of hypervitaminosis A.
- In acanthocytosis, Vit E. is used in doses of 100 mg/wk. intramuscularly and in G-6-PD deficiency it is used in doses of 100 mg/day.

- In conditions like muscle cramps, fibrocystic diseases of breast, etc., Vit. E is used in doses of 400 to 600 mg per day.

Drug interactions

- Prolonged use of liquid paraffin may hamper the absorption of Vit. E.
- Iron absorption may be hampered by concomitant Vit. E administration.

Adverse drug reactions

It is a relatively non-toxic substance. Milder side effects are diarrhoea, abdominal colic and lethargy. A few cases of defective wound healing and creatinuria have been reported.

Vitamin K

It has already been discussed in the previous chapter.

Vitamin B-complex

The important members of this group are thiamine, riboflavine, nicotinic acid, pyridoxine, folic acid and cyanocobalamin. Other members of this group include Inositol, Biotin, Methionine, Choline, Pantothenic acid and PABA (para-amino benzoic acid).

Thiamine (Vit B$_1$)

It is present in outer layers of cereals, green vegetables, peas, beans, pulses, meat, yeasts, etc. Fruits are also good sources of thiamine. The average daily requirement is about 1 to 2 mg.

Physiological Role: It is converted in the body into thiamine pyrophosphate (physiologically active form) and takes part in carbohydrate metabolism by functioning as a coenzyme in decarboxylation of alpha keto acids (e.g. pyruvic acid, alpha ketoglutaric acid); it also takes part in utilization of pentose in hexose monophosphate shunt. For diagnosis of thiamine deficiency, transketolase activity in R.B.C. can be measured.

C/F of deficiency of thiamine

General: Severe deprivation of thiamine leads to Beriberi (dry type, wet type, infantile type). Besides Beriberi, there may be polyneuritis, Wernick's encephalopathy and Korsakoff's psychosis. Deficiency of thiamine in the East in mainly due to consumption of polished rice and in the West it is mainly due to consumption of excessive alcohol.

Specific ocular deficiency features

Thiamine deficiency has been found to be associated with retrobulbar neuritis, conjunctival and corneal hypoaesthesia.

Preparation and dosage

- Tab. Thiamine hydrochloride ranging from 5 to 50 mg; prophylactic dose is 2 to 5 mg per day and therapeutic dose is 25 to 100 mg per day.
- Inj. Thiamine hydrochloride – The dose is 25 to 100 mg given subcutaneously or intramuscularly.

Adverse drug reactions

Thiamine is a non-toxic drug when given orally. But a few cases of anaphylactoid reactions have been reported following intramuscular injection.

Riboflavine (Vit. B$_2$)

The natural sources of riboflavine are green leafy vegetables, whole grain, yeast, milk, egg, meat, etc. The daily requirement in case of children is 0.6 to 2 mg and 1.5 to 3 mg in case of adults.

Physiological role

By the process of phosphorylation, riboflavine gains its physiologically active form. This active form is contained in two coenzymes – flavin mononucleotide (FMN) and flavine adenine dinucleotide (FAD) which play a vital role in hydrogen transfer and in oxidation reactions of carbohydrate and amino acid metabolism. Clinically, cases of riboflavine deficiency can be confirmed by urinary excretion level of riboflavin (it becomes less than 50 microgram per day).

Deficiency features

General: The first signs of deficiency to appear are angular stomititis and pharyngitis. Gradually, features like cheilosis, glossitis and seborrheic dermatitis involving face, body and extremities are evident; ultimately, neuropathy, and normochromic, normocytic anaemia develop. There may be reticulocytopenia. WBC count and platelet count are usually normal. All these features are reversible on administration of riboflavine.

Specific ocular deficiency features

A number of conditions have been described but the most important ocular features are vascularization of cornea (causing distortion of normal vision), cataract formation, SPK like lesions, blepharoconjunctivitis, etc.

Preparations and dosage

- Tablet Riboflavin (2 mg) – Prophylactic dose is 1 to 4 mg per day and therapeutic dose is 5 to 10 mg per day.
- Inj. Riboflavin (10 mg/ml) – The usual dose is 2 to 5 mg per day given subcutaneously or intramuscularly.

Nicotinic Acid (Vit. B_3)

The term niacin is used to denote both nicotinic acid and its amide; and both of them can prevent pellagara but their pharmacological actions differ. One mg of nicotinic acid can be obtained from 60 mg of an amino acid called tryptophan. Hence, tryptophan is also called provitamin of B_3. Maize contains low amounts of tryptophan and so maize eaters are more at risk to develop pellagra. However, pellagra is found to occur mainly in chronic alcoholics, children with protein energy malnutrition and people with multiple vitamin deficiencies. The main dietary sources of vitamin B_3 are fish, meat, chicken, liver eggs, cereal, husks, vegetables, pulses, nuts, etc. The average daily requirement of vitamin B_3 is 15 to 20 mg.

Physiological role and pharmacological actions

Nicotinic acid is converted in the body into nicotinamide which by acting as an important constituent of coenzymes NAD (nicotinamide adenine dinucleotide) and NADP (nicotinamide adenine dinucleotide phosphate) takes part in various oxidation-reduction reactions essential for tissue respiration, fat synthesis and glycolysis.

Nicotinic acid in high doses possesses the property of lowering plasma lipid and property of vasodilatation. But nicotinamide has no such property.

Deficiency features

1. *General*: Deficiency of vitamin B_3 causes pellagra characterized by diarrhoea (with stomatitis, glossitis, salivation, etc.), dermatitis (sun burn type erythematons reaction first appearing on back of hand and then gradually involving other parts of body which desquamate with subsequent scar formation), and dementia (CNS depression sign which in severe cases may lead to hallucinations, delusion, peripheral neuropathy, etc.). Associated biochemical and pathological findings include macrocytic anaemia, hyperuricaemia and hypoalbuminaemia.

Attempts were made to diagnose deficiency of vitamin B_3 by estimating blood niacin level and urinary N-methyl nicotinamide level, but the results were fallacious and so the present day concept is to rely on therapeutic diagnosis.

2. *Ocular*: Many case reports of niacin deficiency have been documented. Some important features are conjunctival irritation, optic neuropathy and macular pigmentation.

Drug interactions

Long continuous use of isoniazide (INH) may inhibit the synthesis of niacin from tryptophan and may lead to development of features of pellagra.

Important preparations and dosages

- Tab. nicotinic acid 50 mg: Prophylactic dose is 15 to 30 mg per day and therapeutic dose is 50 to 250 mg per day.
- Inj. nicotinic acid: It is available as 10 ml ampoules which contain 100 mg of nicotinic acid.
- Tab. Nicotinamide: 50 mg tab.

Adverse drug reactions

Nicotinamide is a harmless drug. Nicotinic acid in large doses may cause flushing, gastro-intestinal upset, activation of latent peptic ulcer, hyperuricaemia, atrial arrhythmia, hepatic dysfunction, precipitation of diabetes mellitus, pigmentary changes of skin, etc.

Pyridoxine (Vit. B$_6$)

Source, physiological role and pharmacological action

It is available in nature as pyridoxine, pyridoxal and pyridoxamine. Pyridoxine and pyridoxamine forms are converted in the body to pyridoxal and then finally they are phosphorylated to pyridoxal phosphate, which is the coenzyme form. Two important pyridoxal-dependant enzyme systems are decarboxylases and transaminases, and vitamin B$_6$ is involved in the synthesis and degradation of various compounds like GABA, catecholamines, etc. Two important reactions which depend on vitamin B$_6$ are conversion of tryptophan to 5-hydroxytryptamine and conversion of methionine to cysteine. It is also involved in the synthesis of various compounds like non-essential amino acids, histamine, aminolevulinic acid, etc. Demand of pyridoxine in the body is dependent on protein intake. Individuals taking 100 g protein/day need 1.6 mg of pyridoxine. The food sources of this vitamin are liver, egg, meat, cereals, whole grain bread and many vegetables. Pyridoxine does not have as such acute toxicity or strong pharmacodynamic action, but consumed for a longer period in doses like 200 mg/day it may give rise to neurological problems like peripheral sensory neuropathy, ataxia, etc. High doses given I.V. have been reported to produce convulsions.

Deficiency features

1. Dermatological lesions like seborrheic dermatis have been found to occur which clear up rapidly on administration of Vit. B$_6$.
2. Convulsive seizures may occur because of pyridoxine deficiency due to low level of neurotransmitters like GABA, norepinephrine and serotonin.
3. Carpal tunnel syndrome associated with a peripheral neuritis has been observed in some cases.
4. Pyridoxine deficient anaemia has been observed which responds to pyridoxine therapy. The anaemia is of hypochromic microcytic type. Vitamin B$_6$ status of the body can be found out by measuring urinary

level of xanthenuric acid (a metabolite of B_6) after giving a full loading dose of tryptophan.

5. Ocular features include:
   - Vascularisation of cornea
   - Optic neuropathy
   - In gyrate atrophy, high doses of Vit. B_6 (more than 20 mg/day) reduce the ornithine level in plasma and the improvement in the clinical condition is evidenced by improved ERG and EOG.

6. In some cases of homocystinuria with downward subluxated lens, pyridoxine level is found to be deficient and administration of Vit. B_6 improves the condition.

Drug interactions

- Isoniazid may induce a pyridoxine deficiency state.
- Pyridoxine utilization can be affected by drugs like hydralazine, penicillamine, cycloserine, etc.
- Levodopa and pyridoxine promote formation of dopamine from levodopa in peripheral tissue. So less amount remains available to reach the specific site of action and ultimately the effect of levodopa in Parkinsonism is not achieved.
- In some females, oral contraceptives may reduce pyridoxal phosphate level and thereby produce mental changes.
- Iron preparations are not utilized properly leading to defective erythropoesis in many cases of pyridoxine deficiency.

Preparations and dosage

- Tab. Pyridoxine: It is available as 5 mg tablet. The usual dose is 5 to 10 mg/day.
- Inj. Pyridoxine: The usual dose is 25 to 100 mg 1.M. or I.V.

Vitamin B_{12} (Cyanocobalamin and Hydroxycobalamin)

Non-vegetarian foods like fish, egg, meat, etc., are rich sources of Vit. B_{12}. In nodules of root vegetables it is present where microbes synthesize Vit. B_{12}. Absorption of vitamin B_{12} is incomplete and so the daily required dose is suggested to be 0.3 mg in infants, 2 mg in adults, and 3 mg in pregnant and lactating mothers. For absorption of vitamin B_{12}, an intrinsic factor (IF) is required, which is a glycoprotein, secreted from stomach. Vit. B_{12} is absorbed from ileum. In plasma, vitamin B_{12} circulates along with transcobalamine II; majority of it is stored in liver.

Important physiological role

Vit. B_{12} along with folic acid helps in the synthesis of DNA and RNA and they maintain the integrity of neurological and haemopoetic system. The normal plasma level of vitamin B_{12} is 140 to 750 pg/ml. Assay of Vit. B_{12} level can be done by microbiological methods utilizing Euglena gracilis or Lactobacillus lechmanii.

Deficiency features

- There is involvement of both haemopoetic and nervous systems. The basic haematological finding is megaloblastic anaemia due to defect in DNA synthesis.
- Early neurological manifestations are diminished vibration sense, disorientation of space diminished tendon reflexes, and paraesthesia of upper and lower extremities. Later on, there are delusion, dementia, hallucinations, visual impairment and frank psychosis.
- The diagnosis of vitamin B_{12} deficiency can be done by examination of peripheral blood smear, gastric function tests, estimations of plasma concentration of Vit. B_{12} and methylmalonic acid level (this is more sensitive), and Schilling test (by which differentiation between primary ileal cell disease and intrinsic factor deficiency can be made), etc.

Some common Vit. B_{12} preparations and dosage

- Inj. Cyanocobalamin – 100 mcg/ml.
- Inj. Hdroxycobalamin – 100, 500, 1000 mcg/ml.
- Tab. Methylcobalamin – 0.5 mg tab.

Adverse drug reactions

Vit. B_{12} is remarkably free from side effects; allergic reaction which sometimes occurs is usually due to preservative or vehicle.

Folic Acid

It is present in green vegetables, egg, milk, meat, liver, yeast, fish, etc. After absorption, the conjugated form of folic acid is hydrolyzed to pteroylmonoglutamic acid, which is absorbed from jejunum. As the absorption is incomplete, the recommended daily intake of folic acid for children is 200 mcg and for adults it is 400 mcg. During pregnancy, the recommended dose is 600 to 800 mcg. Pteroylmonoglutamic acid is converted into tetrahydrofolate (THF) intracellularly with the help of a cobalamine dependant enzyme. At this stage, Vit. C gives protection to this reduced product from being destroyed by oxidative destruction. Total body folate is about 5 to 10 mg of which about 1/3rd is stored in liver. It is distributed to the RBC during erythropoesis and the amount inside them remains fairly constant throughout their life span. So folate level in RBC serves as an important index for diagnosis of folic acid deficiency.

Important physiological role

Along with Vit. B$_{12}$, it helps in the synthesis of DNA and RNA through many biochemical reactions. Serum level of folic acid can be detected by microbiological methods utilizing Streptococus faecalis and Lactobacillus casei.

Deficiency features

General: Megaloblastic anaemia is the common clinical feature. It is not associated with neurological problems unless there is deficiency of Vit. B$_{12}$ also.
Ocular: Folate deficiency may occur while treating a patient with pyrimethamine for toxoplasmosis.

Preparations and dosage

- Tab. Folic acid, 5 mg. The usual prophylactic dose is 0.5 mg/day and therapeutic dose is 2 to 5 mg/day.
- Inj. Folinic acid, 3 mg/ ml injection available.

Adverse drug reactions

It is a remarkably non-toxic drug.

Miscellaneous Members of Vit. B Complex Group

These are inositol, biotin, methionine, choline, pantothanic acid and para-amino benzoic acid. Inositol plays some role in fat metabolism. Deficiency of biotin may lead to alopecia and dermatitis. Choline + methionine is also called lipotropic factor and is used in cirrhosis of liver. Pantothanic acid is converted into coenzyme A which takes part in many vital biochemical reactions.

Vitamin C (Ascorbic Acid)

It is present in adequate amounts in citrous fruits, green vegetables, tomatoes, etc. The daily requirement in the case of children is 5 mg/kg of body weight and in the case of adults it is approximately 30 mg.

Important Physiological Functions

- Concerned with tissue respiration.
- Helps in formation of collagen, intercellular matrix, bone, cartilage, teeth, etc.
- Plays important role in erythropoesis.
- Helps in the synthesis of various hormones like corticosteroid, oxytocin, ADH, etc.
- Maintains the integrity of vascular endothelium.
- Promotes healing of wound like corneal ulcer.

Deficiency Features

- General: The deficiency syndrome is called scurvy, which is characterized by swollen and bleeding gum, anaemia, stunted growth with brittle bones, ecchymoses, petechiae, subperiosteal haemorrhages, etc. Usually, nowadays bottle-fed babies (human milk contains adequate amount of Vit. C), people with peptic ulcer (unable to take citreous fruit), malabsorption disease and patients with severe burns develop features of hypovitaminosis C.
- Ocular: Ophthalmologic manifestation of hypovitaminosis C includes subperiosteal haematoma, retinal, subconjunctival and anterior chamber haemorrhages.

Preparations and Dosage

- Tab. Ascorbic acid is available in 100 mg to 500 mg.
- Inj. Vit. C is available as 500 mg/ml. Prophylactic dose of Vit. C is 25-75 mg/day. Therapeutic dose is 200-500 mg/day.

Therapeutic Use

- For prophylactic therapy in patients and babies who are at risk.
- In the management of scurvy, 0.5-1.5 g per day in divided doses.
- For acidification of urine, 3-4 g per day, as some antimicrobials used to treat urinary tract infection need acidurine, e.g., methenamine.
- Anaemia of scurvy.
- To promote wound healing in post-surgical cases.
- In the treatment of methaemoglobinaemia, but it is not superior to methylene blue.
- Used as antioxidant along with beta-carotene and alpha-tocopherol
- For promoting healing in alkali burn of cornea.
- It can be used as osmotic agent, intravenously to reduce acute rise of tension in narrow angle glaucoma subjects, but I.V. mannitol is superior. For this purpose 250 to 500 mg of 20% sodium ascorbate is infused slowly over a period of one hour.

Adverse Drug Reactions

Prolonged and uninterrupted use of large doses of vitamin C. may cause oxaluria and subsequent renal calculi formation. Infants born of mothers taking large quantities of Vit. C. during pregnancy may develop rebound scurvy.

Antioxidants

Oxidative free radicals are constantly generated in human body during various metabolic reactions, e.g., COX and LOX pathway process, metabolism of alcohol, ultraviolet radiation, etc. These free radicals are either atoms or molecules with one or more unpaired electrons and are highly reactive towards acquiring electrons from other substances. These oxidative free radicals may damage cellular organelles, membrane lipids, nucleic acid, etc.

Epidemiological survey has pointed out that these free radicals are connected with pathogenesis of various conditions like diabetes, cancer and various cardiovascular and neurological diseases. In ophthalmology, such free radicals have been found to be associated with conditions like cataract, ARMD, defect in ocular perfusion, raised IOP and various uveal and retinal inflammatory diseases.

Pharmacological agents used as anti-oxidants are vitamin A, C and E. Other agents include various trace elements (Zn, selenium) and some food articles (fruits, tea, garlic, clove, cardamom, etc.). However, the exact role of antioxidants as pharmacological agents is not yet fully understood.

Recommended Further Readings

1. Carruthers S.G., Hoffman B.B., Melmon K.L., Nierenberg D.W. eds. *Melon and Morelli's Clinical Pharmacology.* 4th ed. New York: McGraw Hill; 2000.
2. Dromer F., McGinnis M.R. et al. In: Annaissie E.J., McGinnins M.R., Pfaller A. eds. *Clinical Mycology*, 1st ed. Churchill Livingstone; 2003.
3. *Drugs: Facts and Comparison.* 56th ed. St. Louis: Walters Kluwer Health; 2002.
4. Gilbert D.N., Moellering R.C., Jr., Sande M.A. *The Sanford Guide to Antimicrobial Therapy* 29th ed. Hyde Park: Antimicrobial Therapy Inc.; 1999.
5. Goyer R.A., Clarkson T.W. "Toxic effects of metals". In: Klaassen C.D. ed. *Casarett and Doull's Toxicology.* 6th ed. New York: McGraw Hill; 2001.
6. Hall A.J. "Differential diagnosis and management of inflammation affecting the retina and/or choroid". In: Lightman S. ed. *HIV and the Eye.* London: Imperial College Press; 2000.
7. Kaufman D.A., Trobe J.D., Eggenberger E.R., Whitaker J.N. "Practice parameter: the role of corticosteroids in the management of acute monosymptomatic optic neuritis". Report of the quality standards subcommittee of American Academy of Neurology. *Neurology.* 2000; 54: 2036-2044.
8. Levy R.H., Thummel K.E., Trager W.F., Hansten P.D., Eichelbaum M. eds. *Metabolic Drug Interactions.* Philadelphia: Lippincott Williams and Wilkins; 2000.
9. Mandell G.L., Bennett J.E., Dolin R. eds. *Mandell, Douglas and Bennett's Principles and Practice of Infectious Diseases.* 5th ed. Philadelphia: Churchill Livingstone, Inc.; 2000.
10. Page C.P., Curtis M.J. et al. eds. *Integrated Pharmacology.* 2nd ed. London: Mosby; 2002.

11. Ramkrishnan S., Prasannan K.G., Rajan R. "Energy metabolism, nutrition, composition of foods and balanced diet". In: *Textbook of Medical Biochemistry.* 3rd ed. Hyderabad: Orient Longman; 2001.

12. Scriver C.R., Beaudet A.L., Sly W.S., Valle D., Childs B., Kinzeler K.W., Vogelstein B. eds. *The Metabolic and Molecular Bases of Inherited Disease.* 8th ed. Vol. 2. New York: McGraw Hill; 2001.

13. Sporn M.B., Roberts A.B., Goodman D.S. eds. *The Retinoids: Biology, Chemistry and Medicine.* 2nd ed. New York: Raven Press; 1994.

14. Sweetman S.C. (ed.). *Martindale, The Complete Drug Reference.* 33rd ed. London: The Royal Pharmacological Society of Great Britain; 2002.

15. Taylor P., Luo Z.D., Camp S. "The genes encoding the cholinesterases: Structure, evolutionary relationships and regulation of their expression". In: Giacobini E. ed. *Cholinesterases and Cholinesterase Inhibitors.* London: Martin Dunitz; 2000.

Index